Raising Benjamin Frog
A Mother's Journey with her Autistic Son

By

Lynne Collier

Raising Benjamin Frog

© 2013 by Lynne Collier. All rights reserved.

No part of this book may be reproduced in any written, electronic, recording, or photocopying without written permission of the publisher or author. The exception would be in the case of brief quotations embodied in the critical articles or reviews and pages where permission is specifically granted by the publisher or author.

Although every precaution has been taken to verify the accuracy of the information contained herein, the author and publisher assume no responsibility for any errors or omissions. No liability is assumed for damages that may result from the use of information contained within.

All scripture quotations are from the "NIV" Bible - the HOLY BIBLE, NEW INTERNATIONAL VERSION®. NIV®.
Copyright ©1973, 1978, 1984 by International Bible Society.
Used by permission of Zondervan. All rights reserved.

Books may be purchased online:

createspace.com

amazon sites

Or by contacting the author at:

LynneCollier.com

lynnecollier@thewhiterosewriters.com

thewhiterosewriters.com

ISBN-13:978-1494443795

ISBN-10:1494443791

First Edition 2013-12-10

Dedication

I wrote this book because I have a story to tell; a story of a mother's love and special bond with her autistic child.

I wrote this book because I was asked to by others who felt my story would encourage mothers whose children are autistic.

I wrote this book because my son is now an adult and I can look back on the years we were growing together and discovering each other's world.

I wrote this book for him. This is *his* story. I was blessed, and still am, to be an observer and a special person in his life.

For Benjamin

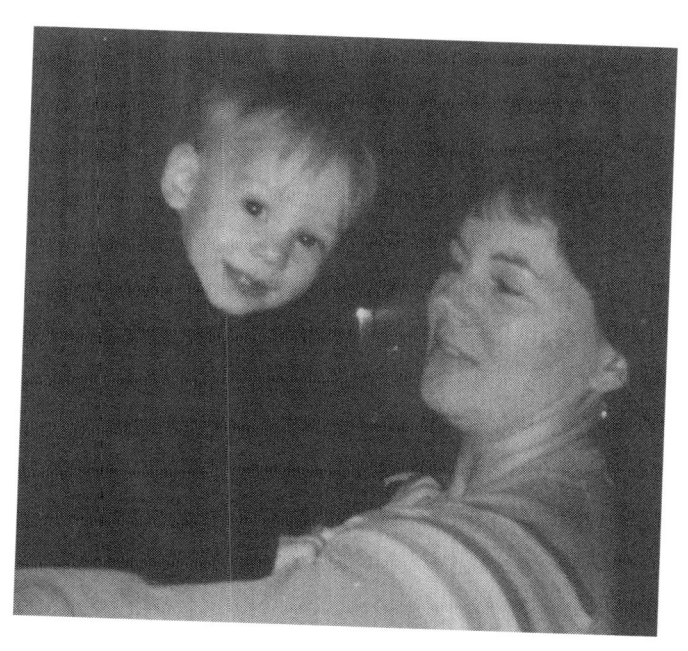

CONTENTS

Acknowledgements
Introduction – A Mother's Cry   13

The Start of The Journey

- Where do you go to, My Sunshine?   15
- The Origin of Benjamin Frog   17
- "Eyes"   19
- Discipline   21

The Formative Years

- Darmok and Jalad at Tanagra   25
- Kindergarten   29
- Stop – Motion   31

The 'Big School' Years

- That's Too Loud!   35
- Falling Down Stairs   37

- Not Quite Michael J. Fox — 39
- Dr. Mary Mac — 41
- Evolution of a Writer — 43
- If you Want to Know What's On... — 45
- Behavioural Mod — 47
- Black and White and Red — 51

Homeschooling

- The River of Knowledge — 57
- The Inquisition — 59
- Thematics — 63
- Amazing — 67
- Some Mothers do Have Them — 69

Photo Album — 71

Acting Career

- "I Want to Do That!" — 87

- Toronto Casting 91
- The Big Screen Years 97
- Everybody Line Up 103

The Teen Years

- The Rescuer 105
- The Young Adult Years 107

Everyone Has a Purpose

- Life Purpose – Mine 113
- Life Purpose – Benjamin's 119

The Journey 123

About the Author 125

Footnotes and Recommended Reading 127

Acknowledgements

A great big thank you to my family. To my husband and life-long journeyer, Stephen; thank you for your patience with me during difficult times and for not giving up on our dream of a happy home for our children and grandchildren. You are my quiet strength.

To Anna, my first born child; thank you for your love and support through this task of writing a story that's sometimes difficult to put into words. Thank you for the long talks on the phone. You are my wise advisor.

To Karen, my second child; thank you for your love and encouragement all the way through this journey. Thank you for immersing yourself in Benjamin's world through play, and drawing me in. You are my calming presence.

To Benjamin, my son; thank you for being the wonderful person you are, for helping me see the potential for this book, for opening my eyes to aspects of God's character which I had overlooked, and for always being a source of joy and laughter, and love.

Dr. Mary MacDonald, thank you for having the wisdom to diagnose Benjamin when other professionals didn't see what I already knew in my heart. Thank you for journeying with us from the beginning and for your continued support and friendship.

Dr. Merry Lin, you were the third person to encourage me to write this book. We both agreed, if God gives us three believers to speak words of encouragement, it needs to be. I told you I wouldn't forget!

I am blessed with so many friends in my life who have helped me write this book. Thanks to all of you for your love and support.

The Start of the Journey

A Mother's Cry

Why, Lord?
Why me?
Why my child?

"Because I have a plan for my Kingdom.

Because I have a purpose for him in My Kingdom.

Because I knew you would be the best mother for him, for My Kingdom.

So help him find his purpose for My Kingdom and don't forget,

He's My child - and so are you".

This book is written straight from my heart, about my son. It's the journey of the life we shared as he was growing up; the struggles and the triumphs. It's not a book meant to explain a lot of psychology of the non-neurotypical mind. Nor is it a How-To book about the best ways to teach an autistic child about the foreign world around them. It's simply from the mother of an autistic child. I'm compelled to write it because I know, by God's grace, it will bring a smile to your lips and a tear to your eyes and we will both be blessed by its writing.

"For I know the plans I have for you," declares the Lord, "plans to prosper you and not to harm you, plans to give you hope and a future. Then you will call upon me and come and pray to me, and I will listen to you. You will seek me and find me when you seek me with all your heart." Jeremiah 29:11-13

"You saw me before I was born and scheduled each day of my life before I began to breathe. Every day was recorded in your Book!" Psalm 139:16

Note: You will notice that I've divided this book into many smaller chapters. I did this because, if you're the mother of an autistic child, chances are you only have enough time to read that much at one sitting.

Where do you go to, my Sunshine?

You have the most beautiful blue eyes, my handsome baby boy. Why can't I see you behind them? Where do you go when your eyes wander away from me?

I hold you in my arms and stroke your tiny face, run my fingers through the yellow strands falling across your brow and I search for a glimpse of soul connection, but you are nowhere to be found.

If I let go of your small hand you'll run away or you'll walk in an endless straight line and not care where you're going. You won't see the people on the path in front of you or the tree that blocks your way. You won't run excited to play with the other children on the swings because they're not there in your world.

We walk by the lake. I point at the birds, gracefully gliding, skimming over the lapping waves. A young puppy barks and, for an instant, I see a puzzled frown on your tiny forehead, then it's gone.

I show you the delicate, colourful blue petals of the Forget-Me-Not and we stop for a while to listen to the rustling of the birch. But you walk where I walk and stop when I stop only because I hold on tightly to your little fingers so you don't slide down the bank and disappear. You have no response to these wonders around you.

I tell you how God made all these things. How He loves you and created you as part of His masterpiece too. How you have a purpose in this life and how I'll do my best as your Mummy to help you find that purpose He has planned for you. But you don't seem to hear a word. You just stare into the distance.

We walk back on the path and I sing to you "Forever Young." You don't sing along or dance in circles around me giggling. But oh how I love you my Sunshine.

Where do you go to, my sweet baby boy, when your eyes wander away from me and you're lost in your autistic world?

The Origin of Benjamin Frog

For a long time, Benjamin was called 'Baby' by everyone in the family. So he referred to himself as 'Baby' too. With two older sisters doting on him, the name stuck through most of the toddler stage. When he wanted anything, he would point to it and say *"Baby"*, and his sisters would, of course, get it for him.

As Benjamin got older he started to realize that his name was no longer 'Baby' but now 'Benjamin'. However, I wasn't having much success teaching him his surname. When I would ask him his name I'd get an odd look as if I didn't know what his name was anymore. He'd say *"Benjamin"* but he wouldn't say his surname. Instead, seeing as I was persistent that he have another name as well as Benjamin, he decided that his last name would be 'Frog'. I've no idea why. He doesn't even remember why. It was just what he chose for whatever reason. I've often wondered if it's because, even at a young age, he realized he was 'different'.

Just know that, when he had his first science fair at school, we avoided the frog-dissecting table!

It still sticks to this day. Even though he's known for a long time now that his name is Benjamin Collier, what does he go and call his blog site?

benjaminfrog.wordpress.com

Note: Benjamin's sister, Anna, found this in her notes from her university class on Children's Literature; - on 'Liminality'…
"Frogs are very liminal creatures. They exist on the threshold between two worlds; part of both, part of neither."

"And they admitted that they were aliens and strangers on earth".
Hebrews 11:13b

"Eyes"

When Benjamin was very young he didn't communicate much at all. He simply did as he was told, as much as he knew to do so. We would use single words to tell him "sit", "stand", "walk", "washroom" etc and he would do it. Questions were met with no response, but we talked to him in complete sentences when we were having a one-sided conversation with him; as if he understood everything, in hopes that someday he would.

If we needed a response from him or he just 'wasn't with us', we'd say his name and tell him to "Stop". Sometimes it took several attempts and louder voices but eventually he'd stop. Then we'd walk over to him and hold his head until our eyes were directly in line with his and say, "Look at my eyes". Once we had his focus on our eyes, he seemed to understand that we wanted to talk to him and he listened. After a while, we simplified things and just said, *"Eyes"*, and he would stop and look at us.

By doing this, we were trying to make a connection between our world and his; a way for him to see us and to step into our world for a short time to hear something important. We would do this, for example, when we needed to do something potentially dangerous like crossing the street. We would say, "Cars. Hand", and he would hold our hands and cross the street. Without this strategy, Benjamin was prone to walk in straight lines regardless of traffic, people or brick walls. So this technique was, I believe, a linking of souls which otherwise wouldn't be able to communicate in typical ways.

We tried not to abuse this time because we came to realize that these times in our world were stressful for Benjamin and he was only happy and calm when he was in his own world, but it allowed us, ever so slowly, to connect with him more and more. Benjamin was about three years old when we adapted this technique. Over time he responded easier, calmer and more frequently.

"Eyes!" became a link between two universes; ours and Benjamin's.

Note: Benjamin always gave me 'Good Night' kisses, even when he didn't know why. He just knew they made me happy and for whatever reason, that was important to him. Thank you, Benj, for all the kisses.

Discipline

How do you discipline a child who doesn't understand right from wrong or even what you're saying?

When he was a toddler I would discipline Benjamin as I had my daughters before him, by short sentences of explanation and removal of the offending object, or them. I didn't like corporal punishment but back then it was the accepted form of discipline until a child was old enough to reason with.

Around two and a half to three years old, Benjamin became increasingly more difficult to handle. He was bigger and faster and intelligent enough to get into mischief when I was busy. I knew he didn't always understand my words and the "Eyes" hadn't become an accepted way for him yet, so things were getting 'hairy'.

I shouted the usual *"Don't"* and *"Be careful"* but to apparently deaf-by-choice ears. He was running around the kitchen, through the living room and down the hall and back again with increasing velocity. I knew something was going to get broken, a wall, a glass or a head!

I yelled, *"Don't run in the house, you'll knock something over!"* a couple of times, then I heard the crash. A drinking glass hit the floor and smashed into pieces. I was frustrated with the mess, the lack of time I had right then to clean it up and this child who caused it! I decided to do the old approach of 'spare the rod and spoil the child' and smacked his bottom.

This was a new experience for him and very confusing. He looked at me, looked at the mess on the floor and a puzzled look came over his face. He looked back at me and turned around to see what had happened to his bottom, then back at me again. It was obvious that my actions held no meaning for him. My explanation of the event meant nothing. I cleaned up the mess and decided that other measures would have to be taken to discipline my son.

Plan B: I decided to stand in front of his 'race track' next time he ran a lap around the kitchen. I knew that he would have to stop when he bumped in to me until he processed the situation and changed his route. Once he had stopped I said *"Eyes. Hand"* and I led him away from the broken glass. Once engaged safely in a new activity in the living room, I was able to clean up the mess and carry on cooking dinner. We employed this new technique to future disciplines and avoided a lot of frustration, bumpy heads and broken glasses!

Note: Even if the child doesn't understand in their head, they'll understand in their heart. After all, 'discipline' is the beginning of the journey of 'discipleship' and that's written on everyone's heart.

"Train up a child in the way he should go and when he is older he will not depart from it." Proverbs 22:5-7

The Formative Years

Darmok and Jalad at Tanagra

When other children were watching '*Sesame Street*' and singing nursery rhymes, Benjamin was lining up dinosaurs on the kitchen floor, paying no attention to the world of children on the screen. He had no interest in TV shows or anything else that required any amount of time in one place for very long.

I used to sit him down on my knee on the floor and rock him in time to the music but he'd squirm himself free and wander off. He didn't even bother to speak. No, "Why are you doing that, Mummy"? He just got up and left the awkward situation he found himself in that didn't have a place in *his* world.

I'd put the Care Bears movie on and sing, '*You Are My Shining Star*', as he ran around the room making strange sounds, arms flailing. There was no response to hugs and kisses but he accepted them as part of his day. I sang to him as he ran around and hoped that someday he'd remember the words. The breakthrough came when he discovered '*The Hobbit*' animated movie.

I'd rented it for his sisters to introduce them to the writings of J.R.R. Tolkien. Benjamin sat longer than usual that day as he watched the images on the screen and started humming the songs from The Shire. He was particularly fascinated by the dragon and the chants of the goblins. Sometime later I found him imitating the march of the goblins and chanting. He was interacting!

He was four years old at this time and he wasn't interested in preschool shows or preschool music. He completely skipped that part of childhood. Instead, he jumped ahead about four years and took a liking to, shall we say 'inappropriate for four-year-olds' shows such as '*Monty Python*'! He started saying more words around this time and could label everyday things well enough to communicate his basic needs, but he couldn't communicate his feelings until one day…

We were in the grocery store when Benjamin pointed to a chocolate bar. I said *"Not today"* and the usual frown came over his brow, but this time, he wasn't staring off into thin air. His frown was focused on the chocolate bar. His face showed definite confusion as he stared at the chocolate bar and back again at me. He wanted the chocolate bar but he couldn't get the chocolate bar. To my absolute horror and astonishment he looked at me and said loudly,

"You parrot-faced wazzle!"

Several people nearby looked on, astonished at the words coming out of the mouth of this angelic little boy. I was totally mortified until I suddenly broke out in a wide grin –

My son was communicating his feelings!

He'd used a scene from *Monty Python* where someone had expressed what they were feeling, (frustration and injustice) with those words, and here was Benjamin using those same words to express what *he* felt, (frustration and injustice over the chocolate bar!). I was so happy! He'd made a breakthrough! He'd seen someone else express an emotion this way and then used it to express *his* own emotion! I didn't care at that moment that half the store was staring disapprovingly at this mother's obvious joy over her son's 'rude' behavior. My son was –

Communicating!

Within a few weeks we had all learned to accept the odd replies we'd get from Benjamin when we asked him a question, and the strange questions he'd ask us, using lines from TV shows. We learned to apply these to *his* life, *his* needs, *his* thoughts and *his* feelings.

Benjamin had taught us to communicate with him!

"Hello, little one. You **Are** My Shining Star!"

Note: I'm glad I didn't stop him watching the same shows as his sisters. If I had, the rest of us may never have clued in to his unique form of communicating. It would be several more years before Benjamin learned the English language well enough to hold a conversation and many more years before he finally understood emotions. All of us are uniquely created and often miss the special ways someone else may be trying to let us into their world.

Thank you John Cleese, Eric Idle, Terry Gilliam, Graham Chapman, Michael Palin and Terry Jones of *'Monty Python'*.

Several years later, *'Star Trek; The Next Generation'* used this form of communication in an episode titled *'Darmok and Jalad at Tanagra'*.

Kindergarten

I was hoping that Benjamin's interview for Kindergarten would go a little better than it did. The teacher read over the intake form and her frown grew deeper with every answer on the page. "Benjamin's favourite movie is '*The Hobbit*'? "She asked in amazement. "*Yes*", I replied, quite matter-of-fact. It was the one he sang to!

She showed Benjamin a series of picture cards and asked him what they were. He got most of them right but one of the pictures really stumped him. When the teacher showed me the picture I laughed out loud. It was a picture of an iron. Of course he had no idea what it was! He'd never seen one! I did the ironing late at night when I knew he'd gone to sleep. Ironing with him racing around the room was *way* too dangerous.

The teacher had a struggle with Benjamin the whole of that first year. He wasn't keen on her either. She made him sit still 'for no reason' and he couldn't play with what he wanted to play with, only what she told him he could play with, and he had to play with things he didn't want to play with. When I went to England to visit relatives for a couple of weeks without Benjamin, the teacher told my parents, who were looking after him, that he was much better behaved without me. She suspected that I wasn't raising him in his best interests. When I returned and was told this I asked Benjamin if he had behaved better for the teacher while I was gone. He said he hadn't been good, he'd been sad because I wasn't there.

He wasn't 'behaving better'. He was just sad. You can't squeeze an autistic child into a neurotypical box. Something has to give. Benjamin wasn't a 'fit' for her programmed class. The stress showed on both their faces by the end of the day.

During this time, I was doing home-daycare to help with the family finances. I'd had several children in and out of care since Benjamin was a toddler. I finally decided to work with an agency and they asked if I'd be willing to care for a baby girl with Down Syndrome. I had an interview with the mother and we seemed to fit well, so we took Melanie into our home while her parents worked.

Benjamin was delighted with Melanie and often stood staring at her. She was a delightful child with a loving nature. Benjamin seemed to attract younger children. He told me later that it was because he didn't wear 'masks'. Young children, he said, have a God-given distaste for hypocrisy.

Benjamin gave Melanie the toys that dropped out of the crib and would pat her gently when she fussed. We had Melanie in our home for over three years until Benjamin went to school and it became apparent Melanie needed more social interaction. Because Benjamin was displaying autistic traits but was yet undiagnosed, I hadn't taken other children in. Melanie had needed heart surgery and extra care during recuperation so I had decided the two children were enough for me to care for at the time.

Melanie was almost three and not walking, but would follow Benjamin around the room, crawling. Together they giggled and crawled across the living room and through the kitchen. One day I found them curled up together in front of the radio and Benjamin was singing along to *'Stand By Me'*. He sang it to her every time it came on the radio. We still call it Melanie's song.

Stop-Motion

So, my 5-year-old son wants to be a movie producer!

Where do I start?

I had no idea if this was even a possibility with Ben having autism, but if that's what was in his heart then we'd follow that as far as it would take us, with God's blessing.

Ben had a plethora of figurines, mostly dinosaurs at that time, so I thought that would be a good place to start. I knew a little about Stop-Motion Animation from watching documentaries about making shows like *'Gumby'*. That looked like the easiest and safest approach to helping Ben make his first 'movie'.

I showed Ben on the VHS how each movement on the screen was made. We borrowed a book from the library about flip-page stick figures and how each drawing followed the last to become a continuous story. We practiced some of our own until he understood the concept. Then we rented a video recorder from the local 7/11 store.

When he was ready, Ben lined up his dinosaurs and we started his first movie production. Patiently, he moved his 'actors' just a fraction at a time, changing their arms and legs and the direction they were facing. It was amazing to me how patient he could be when he was focused on something that was important to *him.* Most things he'd done in his life so far were because he *had* to do them for someone else. They were important to the other person but not to *him.* Other people's important stuff was just an infringement into *his* time. Time that he could be making movies!

I don't know how long we took to make the movie. We only had the video recorder one day, so I assume we painstakingly worked away all day until the movie was to Ben's satisfaction. We edited, rerecorded and checked every last detail until I saw the smile on his face. It was finished.

Benjamin was a movie producer!

The story was short, of course, and not too family-friendly. As I recall, many lesser characters were eaten in the making of the movie. But it was a great accomplishment for a young autistic boy with the ambition to become a movie producer. We were both very proud of our work, (I being the assistant producer. Yes, I got a title). We showed the movie to anyone who didn't mind dinosaurs getting massacred.

The movie lasted all of two minutes but it's what's remained since then that's priceless.

The 'Big School' Years

That's Too Loud!

Another common characteristic of people with autism is their sensitivity to loud noises. Benjamin came home from school one day with a note saying he had to be removed from the school bus. Apparently, he had been yelling and when the driver asked him to quiet down he just covered his ears and screamed louder. When I asked Benjamin about the incident he told me the other children were being too loud and it hurt his ears. He shouted at them to be quiet but they got noisier so he covered his ears.

I noticed early on that Benjamin was sensitive to loud noises, such as the train, heavy traffic and babies crying. It's funny how these noises hurt his ears but *he* could yell at the top of his lungs and it didn't bother him. (There are many clinical studies which corroborate this sensitivity in people with ASD). So I had to drive him twenty minutes to school and back from then on.

Then another note came home with him. He'd been pulled from the auditorium during a musical concert. He had been, once again, shouting and crying because the noise hurt his ears. Apparently, he calmed down when he was removed and sat for an hour out in the hall. Great! That's what he wanted, to be removed from the noise! I told the teacher I would keep him home next time there was a concert and play music for him at home. After all, I was hoping music appreciation was what they were going for, not the solitude of a child with sensitivities.

Falling Down Stairs

"Benjamin has difficulty paying attention in class and often disrupts the other students" – Grade One report card.

Well that's because the only time the other children really paid any attention to Ben was when he made them laugh. Making friends was difficult for an autistic 5-year-old. It was the only means of communication he knew that worked at the time.

"Why do you do silly things in class, Benjamin? You know it gets you into trouble".

"Because it makes the other kids laugh".

"Why do you want to make them laugh?"

"So they feel good. I feel good when I laugh".

I got another call from school. He'd been walking into walls and bumping into things again. It had been going on for a few days and his teacher thought he may need his eyes examined, but I knew differently…

We had to pick up some registration forms from the Community Centre. There was a large staircase in the lobby with lots of people around. As we head down the stairs Benjamin played with his dinosaurs on the rail. I was watching the people on the upper level, when suddenly there were frantic shouts from the lobby. I turned around just in time to catch a glimpse of Benjamin's coat cascading down the stairs, his backpack flying and shouts of,

"Oooooh, Aaaaagh!" as he made sure he hit every step on the way down. Everyone stared in utter astonishment; sure that he had broken bones or a concussion. Reaching the bottom, Benjamin jumped up triumphantly with a loud,

"Ta da!"

I just smiled and shook my head. What he *had* was an *audience*!

I found that I needed to take the time to really listen and watch. Only then could I truly understand what he was 'saying'.

Note: This was the start of Benjamin's interest in acting. I had just signed him up for classes before 'The Fall'.

"I'm very good at delivering a punch line at the time it will be funniest. The problem is that I haven't yet learned to keep my mouth shut when someone is eating or drinking" (1)
- Benjamin

Not Quite Michael J Fox

'Back to the Future' was a great hit at the time and it became one of Benjamin's favourite movies for a while. He still has the trilogy in his collection. The interest in the movie sparked a creative bug in Benjamin to produce his second movie.

The timing was right to make this movie while visiting his grandparents in Florida. Benjamin meticulously gathered all his props and enlisted family members to star in his blockbuster.

The biggest challenge was to create a vehicle. We were away from home so the only 'vehicle' available was his grandmother's three-wheel bike with a shopping basket on the front! Benjamin was undaunted. Off he pedaled down the road in the mobile home community as fast as he could - hoping to reach 88 miles per hour! (For those of you who are new to *Back to the Future*, this is the speed at which the DeLorean hits the time portal).

So how exactly do you make a three wheel bike disappear? Simple, you yell "Cut" and stop the film until the star has pedaled around the corner. It actually worked quite well! On the finished movie, Benjamin disappeared and reappeared several times. Everyone played their part according to the producer's directions and Benjamin received accolades for the finished movie. Watching him peddle around the block proved to be the day's entertainment for the other residents too!

Lame as the acting was, we all encouraged Benjamin in his dream and delighted in his ability to focus on something that was important to him. Encouraging him to pursue what he was interested in enabled him to grow into the man he was meant to become. He learned, instinctively, to follow his inner calling; to hear God's voice.

At the time of writing this, Benjamin is still not a famous producer, but I have a suspicion he's still working on that!

Dr. Mary Mac

"Today we're going to see a new doctor. Her name is Dr. MacDonald".

"Can I have fries?"

"We're not going to McDonald's. We're going to see a doctor. Her name is Dr. MacDonald".

"Does she have fries?"

"No".

"What does she have?"

"She's a doctor. She doesn't have food there".

"I want fries. Can we go to the other McDonald that has fries instead?"

(It was obvious this wasn't sinking in).

"Sure, after we see the doctor".

I explained the conversation to the doctor and asked if she would mind if Benjamin called her Dr. Mary Mac, so he wouldn't be confused. She very graciously agreed. She is a wonderful, kind person with a lot of patience.

Benjamin and I went to McDonald's for fries after.

To this day, Dr. Mary MacDonald is called Dr. Mary Mac!

Evolution of a Writer

I watched him as he drew every minute detail of the new creature he'd created. I saw the facial expressions, the anger, the surprise, the horror, reaching from the page. Sinewy arms and legs reached across the story-board, mercilessly fighting another creature more muscular and aggressive; heads will, and do, roll. I felt the Lord prompting me to draw out of my son the imagination that was unfolding on the paper.

"Tell me the story, Benj. What's happening?"

"This guy is killing this guy and they have to go to a different place and then there'll be more monsters to fight".

I noticed the puzzled look on his face. He couldn't comprehend why I didn't understand the story he'd drawn. Usually I seemed quite intelligent! He sucked his cheeks in, (something he did when he was concentrating, and still did well into his teen years), and frowned.

"I can't see the story in your head, Benj. I can only see the drawings on the paper. They don't tell me the whole story in between the pictures. You need to show the 'stuff' that's happening in between".

"How?"

"By writing down some words that say the filling-in parts. Here, I'll show you... Monster #1 killed Monster #2 with an axe and his head got cut off. Then Monster #1 went to another place and killed another monster. How did he get there"?

"On a spaceship".

"Did he kill the other monster?"

"Not yet".

"Tell me".

"The other monster escaped on a big plane and went to a cave on an island".

"That's great! That's filling in the parts in between! Now everyone can understand your story because they can read the in-between words!

An author is born!

If You Want to Know What's On...

Ben didn't like to read or write when he was young. It took too long and required time away from the more important things, like movie-making and drawing.

I was lost for a way to get him to see the necessity of reading. He didn't want to read other people's stories. Why would he? He created his own! Other people's stories weren't nearly as exciting!

The necessity revealed itself one day as I was busy with laundry and Ben had to know RIGHT NOW if *'Harry and the Dinosaurs'* was on the television. I told him I couldn't read the TV book right now because I was busy.

"You can read, Benjamin, so look for today's date in the TV book". (Pause until he finds that. He could only follow one direction at a time at this age). *"Now look for the time you want. What time is it now?"* (Pause till he studies the clock). *"Does it say 'Harry and the Dinosaurs' on the list for this time?"*

"Yes!"

"Ok. You can put it on that channel!"

Note: I used this technique too when he questioned my decisions. He never argued, he just simply asked "Why?" because he wanted to understand why I'd made that particular choice.

It came in handy for steering him (and me!) to God's Word whenever I got frustrated and said *"Because God said so!"* Then Ben would ask *"**Where**?"* and I'd better be prepared to show him which chapter and verse!

Behavioural Mod

After Kindergarten and Grade One at one school, Benjamin was transferred to a second school outside of our school district and had to be bussed there. There he was to receive what was called at the time 'Behavioural Modification'. The School Board said the reason for the transfer was that Benjamin wasn't paying attention in class and was disrupting the other students. They felt that behavioral modification would help to keep him focused. The transfer took three months of red tape.

Benjamin was placed in a smaller class, along with other children who had similar difficulties. I suspect that, today, many of them would be identified on the Autism Spectrum. The children had a daily chart which the teacher would fill in after each class activity. It was to track how the child behaved during the class that day. For each activity completed successfully and on time, the child got a happy face sticker. For any activity not completed, not done according to the curriculum, or for disruptive and inattentive behavior, the child would receive a yucky (tongue sticking out) sticker. For a completed day without any yucky stickers, the child would receive a figurine of a teddy bear. After accumulating a certain number of bears, the child earned lunch out at a fast food restaurant of their choice with one of the teachers. After a certain number of yucky faces, the child would earn a Time-Out in a secluded corner of the room and not be allowed to join in group time or free-play until all the tasks for that day had been completed satisfactorily.

Benjamin continued to bring home daily reports throughout the six months. Comments of "Benjamin does not co-operate" filled each activity page. He would come home from school so despondent every day and head straight to his room. There he played alone for the first two hours after school, until he felt ready to join the family. It took my seven-year-old son that long to unwind after the stress of school. My heart ached for his struggle to just feel like a good boy.

I must add here that I have a lot of respect for teachers past and present. They do the best they can with the rules set before them. Benjamin had a difficult Kindergarten teacher but an amazing Grade One teacher who had an enormous amount of patience for him and all the children in her care. In the Behavioural Modification class, I'm sure the teachers were just as much at a loss what to do to help Benjamin as I was at that time.

However, I soon became unsettled with the negative influence the daily school reports were having on Benjamin's mental and emotional state. The teachers said their hands were tied. Nothing they tried worked in the classroom. They were unable to teach him addition and subtraction as well as reading. I asked what methods they were using but when I offered an alternative to teach him a different way they said they had to teach according to the curriculum set down. The way they taught obviously wasn't the way Benjamin learned. I knew from teaching him basic life skills that his brain wasn't 'wired' to learn the way they taught, but no one could do anything about it.

Benjamin continued to be disruptive in class and be separated from the rest of the children. He missed out on field trips and play activities. I finally asked him why his behaviour was so bad in class and he told me simply that he didn't understand what the teacher wanted. If he knew, he said, he would do it because she seemed sad every time he didn't do it right. He thought she must be sad because she gave him a yucky face every time.

So I resorted to asking the teachers to just send home the work sheets for the day and I would try to teach Benjamin at home according to the way *he* learned and see if that helped. After a long day on the school bus, at school and then unwinding, Benjamin now had to do the entire day of learning as homework. But he did it! He learned after his third attempt to add and subtract. I simply had to explain it a different way until he finally told me he 'got it'.

I had taken the summer before to teach him to read but, at that time, the educational system taught by memorizing and Benjamin didn't develop memory skills sufficiently until he was older. I had taught him by phonics and he was reading Ladybird books at a Grade Two level when he was six years old. When he had gone back to school that year, he fell back into having to memorize and lost his ability to read. So we went back to phonics and he picked it up in no time. That was acceptable to the new school because of the kind of class he was in and they didn't try to teach him reading by memory anymore.

Benjamin also explained to me that he didn't feel bad about being put in the corner away from the other children because it was quieter there and he could use his brain better and no one told him to stop fidgeting because they couldn't see him for the partition.

So I told him not to be concerned about the stickers on his report. If he couldn't go on a field trip that he really wanted to go on we could go together another day, or we could go on a different field trip on that day instead. He got very excited at being able to choose the place himself and just the two of us go, or maybe invite Aunty Debi and her young children because they were nice to him. Then we could do interesting stuff, like pick up rocks and run through the grass. He could take his action figures too. He wasn't allowed to bring them to school. But he missed out a lot on being with the other children and I was glad he went to Sunday School so he could be a part of a group who, for the most part, didn't make him feel like he was bad. I was grateful that our church had wonderful, loving teachers. Benjamin still likes to see his teacher, Mrs. Clyke, and she him, when our paths cross once in a while.

"This life is not a qualifying exam – it's a rehearsal". (2)
-Benjamin

Black and White and Red

During his time in the Behavioural Modification class, Benjamin became self-destructive. He would stab himself on the legs with sharpened pencils. I asked him why and he told me because he was a bad boy and he didn't know how to stop being bad except to stop 'being'. My heart broke. I told him he wasn't a bad boy. He was a very good boy. People who loved him knew what was in his heart, but some other people didn't. I told him I would try to help them to see what a good boy he was.

The turning point in this dilemma came when Benjamin brought home a picture he had drawn at school. Usually, his art was about dinosaurs and creatures he'd made up, and was quite colourful. This particular drawing was about his teachers, himself and his classmates, and was very disturbing. It was in black and white-and *red*!

He had drawn a picture of his teachers and classmates fighting, with guns. Some of them were headless, falling off tall buildings, most of them spurting blood! I was horrified when he showed me the picture! I asked him who the people were and why they were fighting. He still didn't connect with his emotions well at this age so I didn't get a clear understanding of what the problem was. I just knew it was serious. This was not the heart of my little boy.

The next day I called his pediatrician, Dr Mary Mac, and told her about the picture. She immediately scheduled Benjamin for a trip to *Sick Kids Hospital* to see a psychologist and a behavioural therapist. The whole family was asked to go to the initial appointment with the psychologist. Two of us didn't want to go but the psychologist said that she would then assume the problems Benjamin was facing would lie with whoever didn't show up. Everyone went! (Smart doctor).

After two weeks of appointments at the hospital, travelling on the GO train and spending hours in the waiting rooms, the doctors concluded that Benjamin was distraught over the situation at school (really?). They also concluded that Benjamin's school placement should be assessed again. Dr

Mary Mac immediately called the school's principal from her office at *Sick Kids* and told him to halt the daily reports with the yucky faces until a new strategy could be put in place. I had a great deal of respect for her and was very grateful for her intervention.

The difficulty now was that the school board couldn't change Benjamin's behavioural modification programme without a new approach in place. After several weeks Benjamin was scheduled to have an assessment done at the Developmental Centre, again in the city and requiring long days and GO trains. He was to be there for three days and he would be evaluated on Intellectual Development, Social Skills and Emotional Development. So, off we went again to Toronto.

I spent most of the time in the waiting room, talking to other parents of children with difficulties in school, or preschoolers who didn't communicate. Their stories touched my heart and I had a deep sadness for all the misunderstood children and the parents who felt so helpless to care for them.

I was allowed, once, to observe Benjamin from an adjoining room as he was being observed by the medical staff. They were instructing him to place things on the table in order and to group things together. Benjamin just wanted to play with them but I could tell he was trying to cooperate. I was very proud of my little boy, alone in a room with strangers, being told to do things for 'no reason', things that didn't make sense to him, but that I had told him to do anyway and we would go for a treat after.

So, he complied and did his best, but I knew he didn't understand what they were asking him to do. I asked if I could be in the room and explain it so he would understand what was required of him, but that would interfere with the results, they said. So I had to sit and watch as he struggled to conform. I only sat in the observation room the one time.

The results were that the doctors reported that Benjamin was unable to do most of the tasks he was asked to do. I asked if I could explain it 'off the record' and see if he understood. They agreed, just to keep me quiet, I'm sure. I had a feeling I was getting a reputation by this point as a 'difficult mother'. But I explained the instructions to Benjamin as best as I could, according to how I knew he understood, and he completed almost all the tasks. I was overjoyed, and Benjamin was smiling, but it didn't change the results. Benjamin still couldn't follow the instructions if given by anyone else and that's what went on the report.

So Benjamin was sent back into the same classroom with the daily reports and yucky faces and my presence was requested at the Board of Education.

"It is because of me, but it is not my fault."(3)
- Benjamin

Homeschooling

The River of Knowledge

The diagnosis came after Dr Mary Mac asked me how Benjamin's schooling was going. I told her it had been a challenge at first, to realize how Benjamin learned things. I said it was like he was standing on a riverbank and the rushing water was information. The new thing he was trying to learn was on the other side. Other people would find a bridge and cross over to the other side, gathering jars of information safely from the rushing water as they went. Benjamin couldn't find the bridge. All he had were stepping stones of things he'd already learned. If he didn't have the right stepping stone in front of him, he couldn't get to the next stone and the next, and so on to reach the other side. Each new thing he tried to learn had to have an already-learned stone to step onto in order to move forward.

It was a scary and sometimes dangerous place for him, trying to cross the river and get to the other side where everyone else was, while attempting to carry endless jars of information along the way. If it became too scary and he couldn't find a stone in the rushing water, he would sometimes have to turn back. He'd become very frustrated that he couldn't do something other people seemed to find so easy.

From that description, Dr Mary Mac concluded that what Benjamin had was Asperger's Syndrome, a form of high-functioning autism. I had been asking our family doctor about autism since Benjamin was two years old. I was relieved to finally get a diagnosis for him and thought it would help him get the extra assistance he needed in school. She gave me copies of studies and anything else she could find, to try to help me understand my child. I hoped that other people in the family would read it too and learn to understand him. I hoped he'd be able to go back to the 'big' school if he wanted to. I found out most people had already made their own 'diagnoses' of what was 'wrong' with Benjamin. But at least now I knew why he had difficulty and I would learn ways to help him find his stepping stones. Together we would keep holding hands and navigate the river.

The Inquisition

I will apologise here for anyone who was in that room on the day of *'The Inquisition'* who honestly tried to get the best for Benjamin in the public school system and was shot down by bureaucracy.

I sat in the car in the parking lot and prayed. *"God please allow **Your** will to be done in this room today; what **Your** perfect will is for Benjamin, so that he will grow up to be the man **You** created him to be."*

I walked into the room where a group of educational and medical professionals sat in a semi-circle. I was asked to join them at the end of the table. They all had a folder in front of them and I was given one too. Someone from the Board of Education led the discussion and the others were asked questions to support the report.

I was told that Benjamin was very disruptive in class and that he failed to follow directions. They had tested his hearing several times over the course of his two years in public school, including after his initial Kindergarten interview so they knew he could hear. The conclusion was that his behaviour was deliberate rather than medical and that he needed further help with behavioural modification. They decided the best course of action would be to send him to yet another school where the teachers specialized in this sort of behavioural therapy. This was three different schools in three years!

They also strongly suggested that I put him on Ritalin. It would help him to comply better. They wanted to change how my son thinks, feels and creates so that he could *'comply'* with how they thought he should behave. Ok mums, you know what's coming!

I was asked politely if I had anything to say. You betcha! But I remained calm and said that I believed Benjamin could be taught without Ritalin if the teachers would adapt teaching strategies which worked for him at home. I would be more than willing to help the teachers in any way I could to better understand how Benjamin learns and what his 'key' words were to 'compliance'. They declined my offer and suggested that they knew what was best, after all, they were experts and I wasn't. They wanted to change my son's personality, his creativity and, only God knows what else the drug would do to him, to make him manageable in class!

So, I called on the One who created Benjamin and suggested to the group of experts that, while they certainly knew more about education in general than I did, they didn't know this one child as well as I did. I had spent over seven years with my child, whereas most of them had never met him or, at best, had only spent three days with him in a medical centre. I said I had spent not only every day of his life with him but spent a good deal of time in prayer for him. I asked who in that room had prayed for my son...silence.

"Mrs Collier, we realize that you know Benjamin better than anyone else, and we admire your devotion to him, but we strongly believe that the drug will allow Benjamin to be calm in class and make it easier for him to cooperate and learn better. I'm afraid that, without Ritalin, we won't be able to teach Benjamin".

(Read that last sentence again). I replied, "*Ok.*"

During this time I had spoken to someone who was home-schooling her children. She suggested I look into it. I didn't think I was qualified. I wasn't a school teacher. Surely I needed a degree of some sort. I found out that, as long as I had graduated the grade I was teaching, I could teach that grade/subject etc. Many people tutoring or teaching or coaching are simply more educated about that particular topic than the person they're teaching. You need to be a qualified teacher to teach in the public school system, however.

So, I researched the idea. I thought it might work well for Benjamin with the circumstances at the public school being what they were at the time. It would, at least, give him time away from the stress. He could always go back to school later. I told Benjamin about the idea soon after my meeting with the Board. I'd never seen him so happy! He was beaming - yes, *BEAMING,* from ear to ear!

Benjamin finished the rest of the school year without any incidents. He wasn't stressed any more. He was smiling, playful again, engaging. He even managed to get his first bear! The teachers were very happy. I'm sure they thought their hard work with him was finally paying off, but every time I asked Benjamin if he was sure about not going to school, he said a very loud and emphatic

"*YES!*"

Benjamin received one bear during the six months that he was at that school. It came *after* he knew he wouldn't be going back to the *big* school. His favourite teacher, (who was not a full-time teacher in his class, but a special education teacher who came twice a week to observe the children's progress), was so pleased with his accomplishment. She decided to take him out for lunch. She was my favourite teacher too! She 'got' my son.

Thank you, Chris.

<u>Note:</u> Regardless of the challenges we may face in our lives, we are ALL made in God's image. I knew God had a plan for my son's life and I wasn't going to let strangers, no matter how intelligent, choose who my son should become. I was raising him to fulfill his unique purpose for God. No one else, not even me, knew what that purpose was.

At this age, Benjamin was about 4 years delayed socially but 4 years ahead intellectually. This gap increased each year and was about 10 years delayed/advanced by the time he was in his late teens.

"...the damage we can cause by trying and screwing-up is not as great as the good that will never be if we do nothing at all." 4
- Benjamin

"For we are God's workmanship, created in Christ Jesus to do good works, which God prepared in advance for us to do."
Ephesians 2:10

Thematics

When we first started home schooling I read all the home schooling books I could find, and all the programmes offered to home schooling parents. Keep in mind, this was 1990 and there wasn't a whole lot out there. There wasn't a computer in every home in our town yet. The internet wasn't a household word and the web was still on my kitchen ceiling! I eventually found a curriculum from the *Moore Foundation* that I thought would fit us both and I sent away for it. It was adaptable for children with learning disabilities, and Benjamin was still falling into the 'Behaviourally Challenged' category, depending on who we talked to. High Functioning Autism wasn't something known yet in most households.

I joined a local group of home schooling parents who had established a private school and held social days for the parents and children. They had Science Fairs, Sports Days, Play Days, Field Trips, just like a regular school. The parents met regularly to discuss curriculum and share craft ideas and the like. So we went to the local superstore and bought all the paraphernalia we needed to get started: notepads, pencils, crayons, erasers - no yucky face stickers! We were all set.

I told the *Moore Foundation* about Benjamin's challenges and they suggested I teach him by Thematic Units. That way he would be interested in the theme even if the subject didn't interest him. They were always available to help me and make changes to suit Benjamin's needs. I learned a lot from them about teaching him as an individual, more than a student who had to 'get through' the school year. They also suggested I send away for *James Dobson's* books and pamphlets on *Focus on the Family*. I found them extremely helpful and I loved that I was teaching Benjamin according to how God had ordained. There was great comfort in knowing someone else believed God had a purpose for him.

I picked up Thematic Units from the *Wise Owl* and *Mastermind* stores to compliment the basic skills of Math, Science and Language. It wasn't as difficult as I expected to find

Math, Science and Language Skills represented in dinosaur form, his favourite topic for about three years! I became the only mother in our circle of friends who could name all known dinosaurs at the time! We got off to bed early; both excited to be starting this new adventure of learning together.

We started our first day with Scripture and prayer and sat in the office like Benjamin had done at school so he would see that this was a very regular part of his day at home now. We stood in front of the pile of books and I wondered where to start. So I asked the expert, God. He suggested I ask Benjamin, and Benjamin told me he wanted to get the hard stuff (Math and Language) done first so he could enjoy the good stuff (Science and Free Choice).

So that's what we did. We piled the good stuff on the bottom and the hard stuff on top and he worked away at the pile until he'd finished. When it came to Free Choice, he had a list of subjects to choose from which included Art, Physical Activities, Socializing and Field Trips. Every day he worked hard to finish early so he could choose the last subject.

I found that I had to talk him through some things slowly while other things he grasped easily. I had to encourage him constantly that it was ok not to be perfect. Getting a math question wrong was fine, by me, God and the *Moore Foundation* who supervised his progress. I found out later that perfectionism is a common trait in people with autism and that was what had led Benjamin to feel so bad about himself in the Behavioural Modification class.

Over the years of home schooling we spent three on the dinosaur theme and the rest on a newly acquired delight - video games! I wasn't too disturbed about this, mostly because it helped with his fine motor control and his strategic thinking. Both were important at this age and helped him develop a sense of achievement. It took a while, however, for him to be ok with 'dying'. He did, eventually, learn patience this way. A social aspect of gaming was that it allowed him to play against someone (the computer) and be ok with them winning. He also learned to be a part of a team, which he found difficult in the neurotypical world. He also came to delight in, not only blowing up aliens and bad guys, but also in rescuing the princess! This would prove very useful in his career later on.

<u>Note:</u> Home schooling isn't for every child, and certainly not for every parent!

In our society too, many families need two incomes to pay the bills and raise their children. So if you're thinking of home schooling, please talk to other parents in your community who are already doing that. If you decide to home school, a network of home schooling parents online and a local support group will be very beneficial. I wish you much success and many happy memories.

For tips on families living with one-income, please visit
annasklar.wordpress.com

Amazing

I'm not very good at doing mazes, so when Benjamin proved to be very fast, I was well, - amazed! In fact, as a young child, he would create his own mazes. They were intricate, with their own stories and surprise traps, in all shapes and sizes. At first I thought he was some kind of genius, until we visited the *Geneva Centre for Autism* in Toronto. There I learned that many children with autism are adept at solving puzzles, especially mazes.

Once again I was reminded of the wonderful way my son's mind worked, quite differently from my own. He saw things in a way that seemed illogical to me but made perfect sense to him. It would seem to Benjamin that *this was the obvious way to go*, while I would walk into endless traps and have to start over, only to get stuck again. I remember his puzzled face, cheeks sucked in and brow furrowed, as I relentlessly went the *wrong* way.

Neurotypical brains, I've learned, tend to reason things out while the brain of a child with autism will envision the end result and follow the path. This may not be the clinical explanation but it's the way I see it and the way Benjamin has explained it to me. I'm just a mother who raised an autistic son and asked him about things I didn't understand. I was amazed on a daily basis at his abilities and challenges, and how he coped with them to learn how to adapt to the neurotypical world around him.

Some Mothers do Have Them

The title to this chapter should read 'Some Mothers do 'Ave 'Em', however, after careful consideration, I realized a great number of readers wouldn't be able to pronounce the title. This was a TV show imported from England during the 80's, and one of Benjamin's favourites. It's about a loveable, whimpy guy and his crazy antics. It was also a favourite of mine and Stephen, and we'd watch it with our friends and all our children. It became a favourite of theirs too, with some translation.

Benjamin had quite a talent for impersonating *Frank,* the main character played by Michael Crawford, and copied his mannerisms and stunts with wonderfully scary dexterity! He could speak with a flawless accent and would entertain us with his impromptu performances. He mimicked the famous "Oooooh", with his finger at the side of his mouth, and the unsteady gait with one arm straight by his side and the other hand gesturing in uncertainty.

I found out about Benjamin's talent one day while driving him and his sister somewhere. He was sitting on the back seat of the car, making the usual noises he often did when his mind was elsewhere, when I caught what he was doing.

"Well, put it in the corner and we'll throw it out in the morning!"

Benjamin had memorized every line from the thirty minute sitcom, along with the voice changes for *Frank and Betty*. I laughed so hard, I had to pull the car over before I ran in to something! This was the first time I had heard him do a complete scene from a show.

Stephen and I were going to see Michael Crawford perform the next month, in Toronto. I decided to film Benjamin doing the famous 'Have a Break, Take a Husband' skit and give Mr. Crawford a copy.

Benjamin collected all his props; he needed pyjamas and a sleeveless vest, (that's what *Frank* wore to bed and this scene was on their second honeymoon), a wig for *Betty* (he used a mop head), and a piece of linoleum, (he settled for a door mat). The scene was set up in his bedroom and I started 'shooting'.

After Mr. Crawford's performance in Toronto, I took the video backstage and asked a security man if he would please give it to Mr. Crawford. He smiled and said he would. I had my doubts, but about two weeks later, Benjamin received a package in the mail from Mr. Crawford, thanking him for the video. He also sent Benjamin an autographed photo.

Benjamin heard Mr. Crawford sing later, when I received the original London performance of *'Phantom of the Opera'* on CD as a gift. Mr. Crawford was the original *Phantom*. I think he was impressed with Mr. Crawford's many talents. I was impressed with Mr. Crawford's kindness to my son, and for helping him see the talent hidden inside of him.

Note: I realize, like most mothers, that the people who I remember most clearly are the ones who were kind to my children. These are the people who spoke into my children's lives and made a difference, often without realizing the impact they'd had to change someone's life.

PHOTO ALBUM

I have a few pictures to share with you. They are snapshots of Benjamin as he grew up. I hope you enjoy the visual journey...

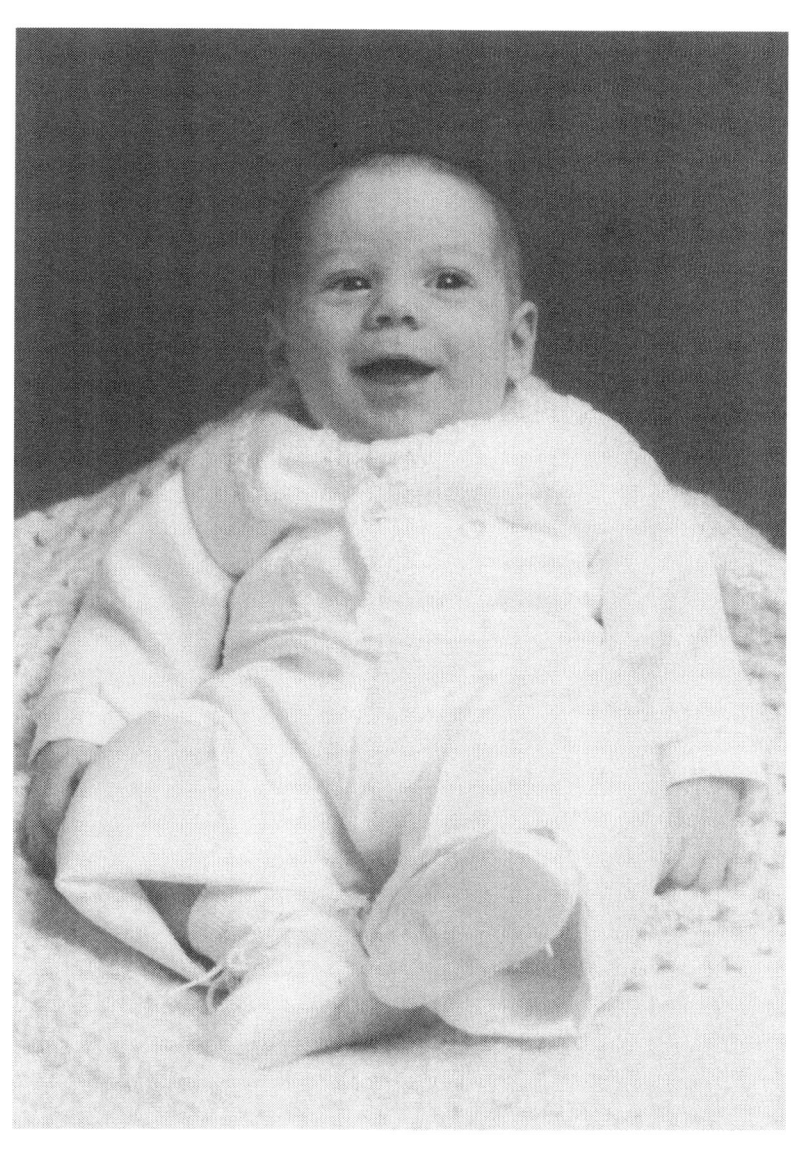

Benjamin's Dedication at 2 months old.

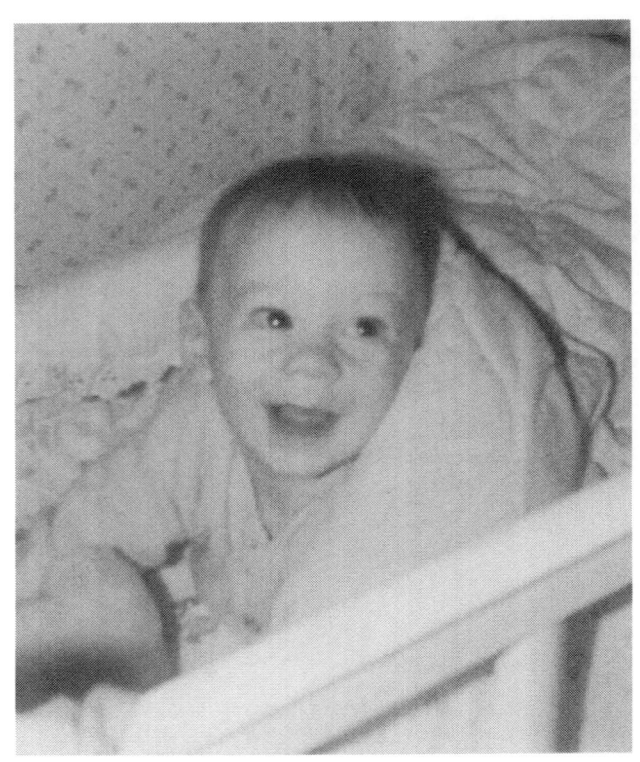

Good Morning, Sunshine!

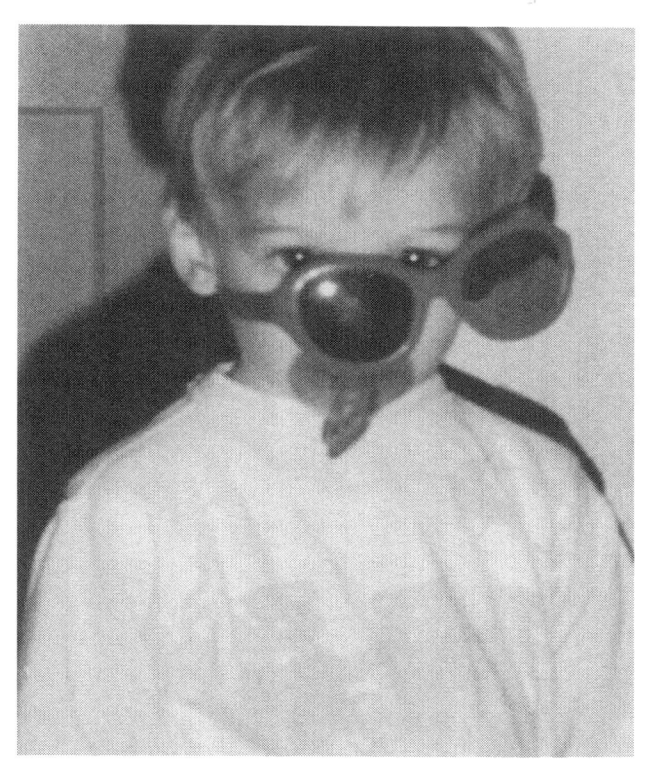

Benjamin's 'Elton John' Look

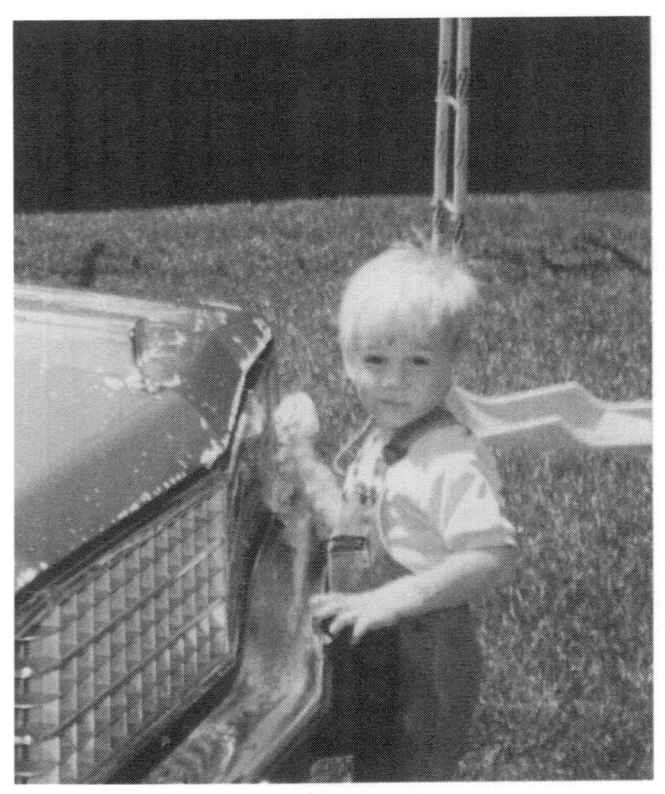

Helping Daddy

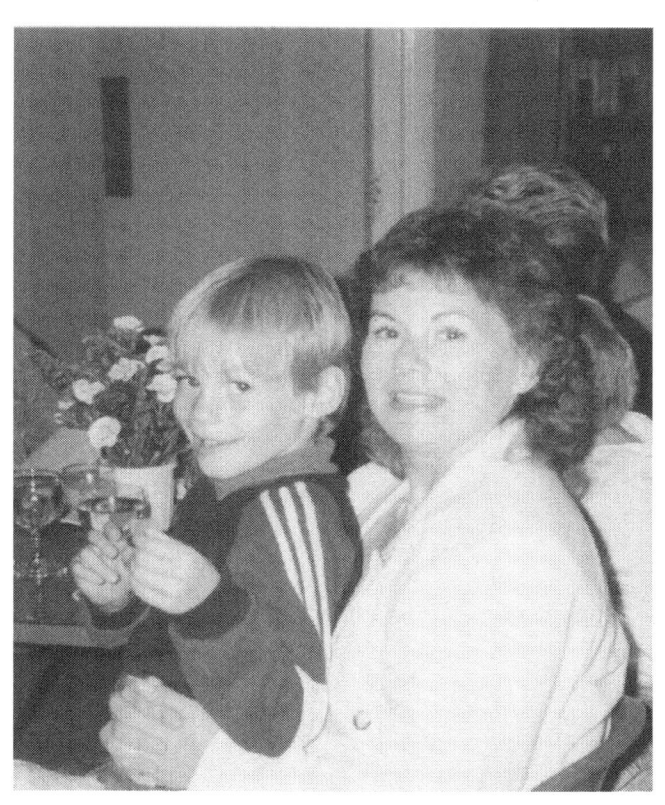

Benjamin at 7 with Mummy

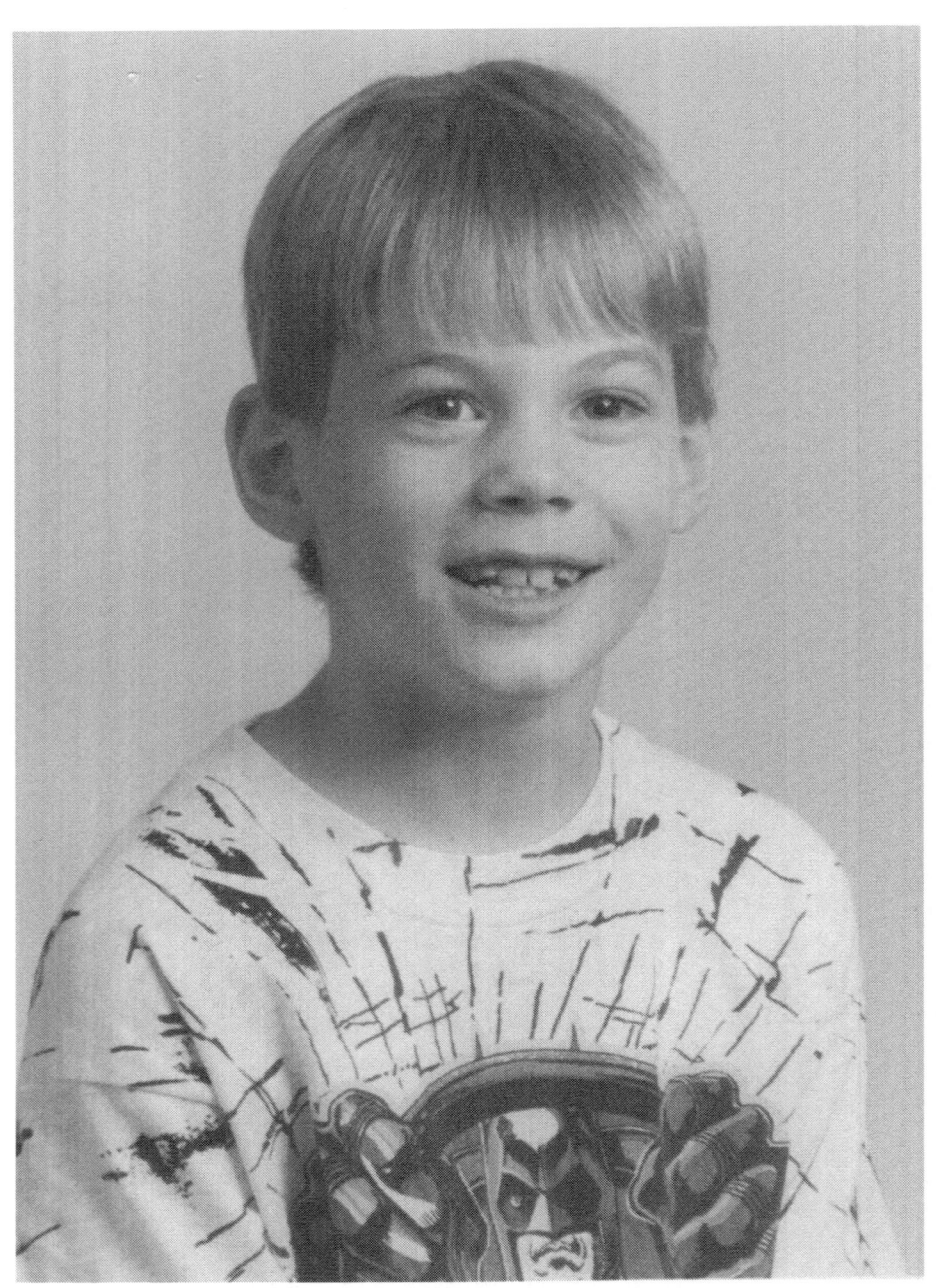
Benjamin's Headshot for Toronto Casting, age 9

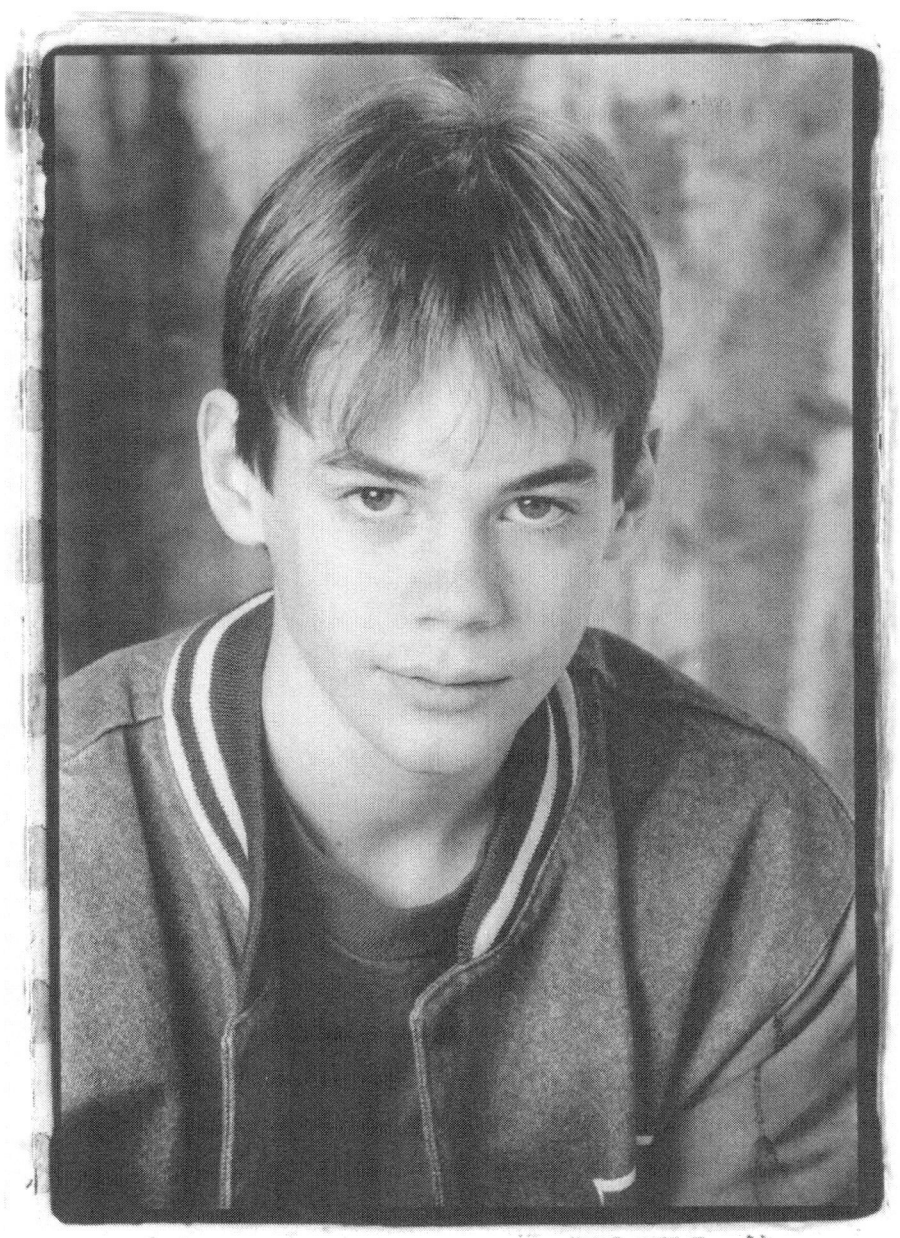

Benjamin's headshot for Toronto Casting, age 14

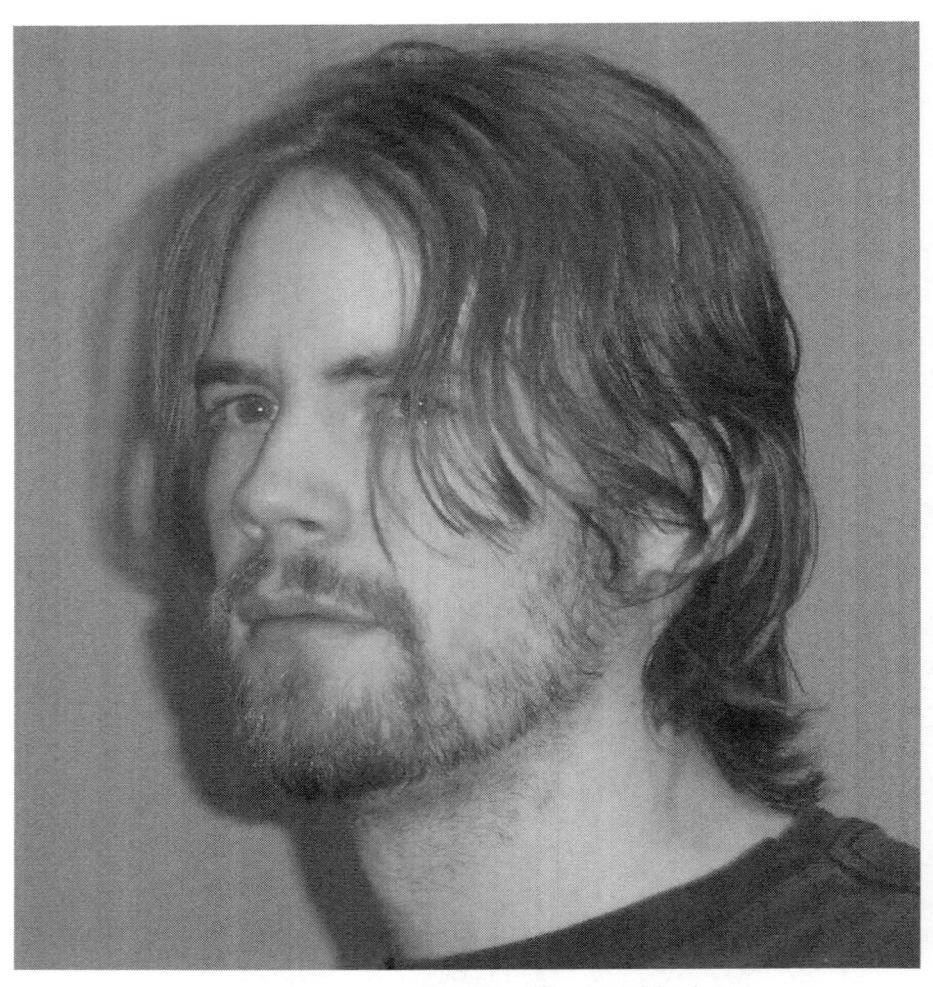

Benjamin at 27, after his 'Sawyer' haircut.

see footnote #6

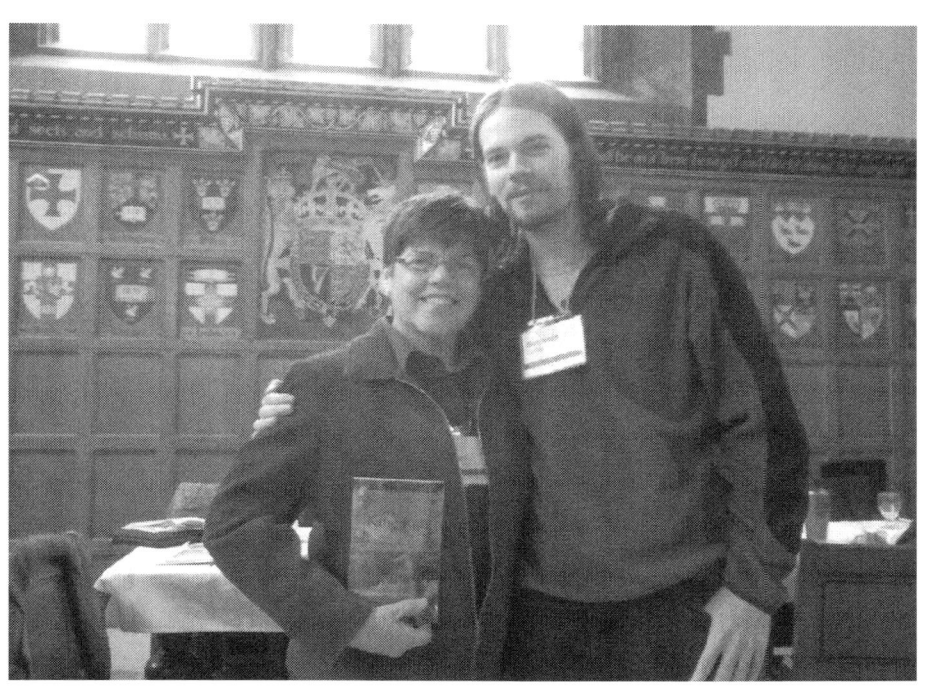

With Dr.'Mary Mac'. Holding his First Book, 'The Kingdom'

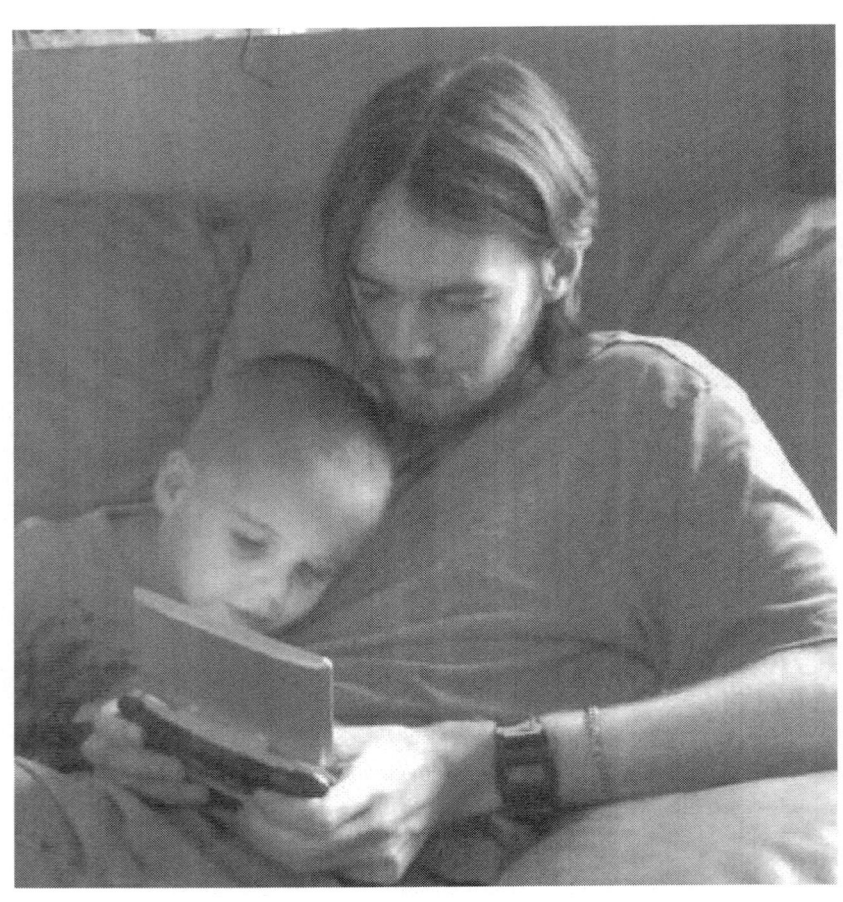

Benjamin with his nephew

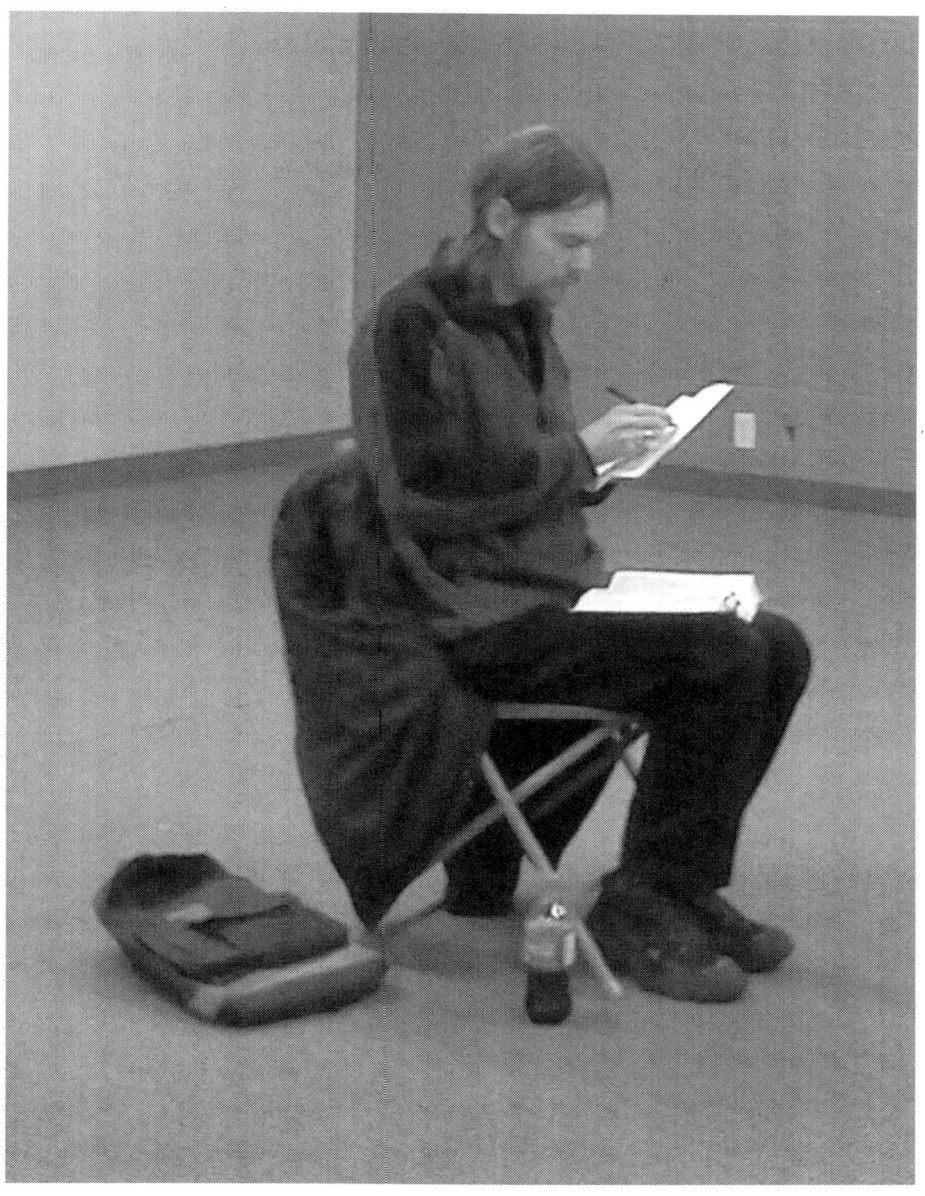

After Alpha
Everyone else had left but Benjamin was still writing notes.
Some of them probably ended up on his blog!

Acting Career

I Want To Do That!

I watched Benjamin as he played in front of the TV. At least now he was interacting with the stories he saw and his sentences were becoming more plausible. He joined in on the action, jumping around and shouting as loud as he could. I wondered, as I often did, what this child of mine would do as he grew up. What were his limitations going to be with having autism? Where would he live? I hoped that he would want to live close to me, at least close enough to visit, but would he be able to live independently? What kind of job would he be able to do? Would he be able to drive? Would he marry? Would he want to?

As I watched him, innocently oblivious that this childhood would end and give way to serious changes, I asked him, *"What do you want to do when you get big?"* (What do you want to be when you grow up didn't 'compute'.) He looked into my eyes to show that he had heard and understood the question, and then redirected his attention to the TV.

"I want to do that!" he exclaimed loudly and pointed to the TV.

"You want to act out the stories like the people on the TV?" I asked him.

"I want to do that!" he shouted again, louder.

I thought to myself, ok he wants to act. Can he do that with autism? He had serious ADHD with the autism too. How was he going to follow directions? He only seemed to be able to follow me and a chosen number of teachers through the years who had patience for him. He saw authority figures as people to dismiss because their rules 'didn't make any sense'.

I decided to look into the possibility of introducing Benjamin to acting. After all, if this was going to be part of God's plan for his life then it was up to me to discover how to actually help him to do that. Would he take direction from someone he didn't know? He had done well with his grade one teacher but not with the teachers at the second school. He seemed ok if the teacher was willing to take the time to explain things in depth, but that distracted the rest of the class. How was that going to work when a director was on a tight deadline and had many other people to direct at the same time? So I enrolled Benjamin in an acting class at the local community centre. If he couldn't do *that* then he couldn't 'do that'.

The night before he was to start classes, I explained to him what he would be doing the next day. This was our nightly ritual, and was through his teens too. He could then go to sleep thinking about the next day and, at least on this night, he could sleep with excitement, thinking about 'doing that'.

The class was held at an old community centre. When we arrived at the class I showed Benjamin where he needed to put his coat and where he needed to sit, and then I explained to the teacher about his autism. At this time there was very little the public knew about autism and his teacher had never heard of it before. She assured me that he would be fine and she would keep an eye on him for wandering off. Miss Linas was a wonderful young girl and helped put my mind at ease. Remember, this was before cell phones, so once I'd left Benjamin I had no contact with the teacher.

When the hour was up, I nervously went to the front door to get Benjamin. There were children everywhere, running around and laughing. I saw Benjamin playing with the other children. He was happy! That was a good sign. I asked Miss Linas how Benjamin had done. She smiled and without hesitation beamed, "Wonderful! He listened to direction. I only had to repeat myself twice for him and remind him of 'eyes' when he wasn't focused. He got along with the other children, as you can see, and they all had a great time! He's a wonderful story teller".

Wow, Benjamin *could* take direction from a stranger, if I told him the stranger was ok and if he was interested in what he was doing! I watched him running around, giggling. He had become part of the group so naturally. My son had found his 'calling' without any direction from me. He had listened to God and obeyed. It was something he was interested in, his natural gifts from God, and something that God knew he could do, even when I doubted.

    Benjamin finished the eight week course without any complaints about going to classes. He even seemed to make friends with a few of the other children there. So I decided to contact a children's acting agency and take it to the next level.

<u>Note:</u> Thanks going out to Miss Linas for her patience and care of Benjamin when he was in her beginners acting class. Because of her diligence, Benjamin later became an 'extra' on many TV shows and movies and the 'creatures' she lured out of Benjamin would go on to be immortalized in print!

Toronto Casting

I found an acting agency which would audition inexperienced children and get them work as background extras to give them practice for future roles in movies and on TV. I called the office and told them a little about Benjamin. I only went as far as to say he had ADD but that he really wanted to act and I felt he would be able to follow directions because he'd recently been enrolled in an acting class. The person on the phone sounded pleased that he'd had acting classes, so I thought we had a chance. She asked if we could come in to meet the agency director the following week. A few days later I told Benjamin I'd booked an appointment to see an acting lady who could help him 'do that'. His eyes widened as I told him about the trip to Toronto on the GO train and how we would have lunch after in the city.

The night before the interview we packed his bag together. This was our usual time to decide what we would do the next day, so that Benjamin would have time to reflect on the coming event and nothing would be unplanned, as much as possible. He didn't adapt well to last-minute changes and always needed time to think things through carefully. If he thought something may not go right, he'd ask me what would happen 'if', and we'd talk it through until he was satisfied that all the possible scenarios had been covered. We packed his new note book we'd bought for him to write and draw about the day, plenty of coloured pencils and erasers, several Transformers, granola bars and drinking boxes. He didn't have a Game Boy yet. He went to sleep without any trouble with a big smile on his face.

The train ride was always a concern. Benjamin still had no fear of trains, traffic or getting lost. This was going to be an ordeal but one, I hoped, that would lead to a future career, as much as he was able, in a field he was growing more and more interested in each day. He was still only eight years old. We could take our time. The first troubling part came when I had to pay for the GO train tickets. I had to hold tightly to Benjamin with one hand and fumble with my wallet with the other. He tried to wander off a few times as we waiting on the platform. I was beginning to wish I'd brought the walking bracelet. I'd used one many times before when we went for day trips to Toronto or anywhere where there would be a crowd and risk of him getting lost. It tied his wrist to a plastic rope and then to my wrist. I was hoping I wouldn't need it today because he was excited to do what we were setting out to do. I took him to the waiting shelter so he could occupy his mind playing with his Transformers. Waiting on the platform was about to raise my blood pressure!

As the train approached the bell began to ring loudly. Benjamin crouched down, covered his ears and put his head between his knees. Once the train stopped he looked in amazement at this big machine in front of him. He'd been on the train before but not very often. The rest of the day was all going to be new things. I was nervous and at the same time totally elated at the adventure.

"Let's find a seat where we can see the lake, Benj".

Benjamin had other ideas, of course. He chose to go upstairs to the top floor and sit by the stairs, in the alcove seats. He later explained that he did this so he could escape if things didn't go well. He always felt better when he knew he didn't have to stay somewhere if it became frightening to him or he felt at risk.

Here, in the seats by the stairs, he played with his Transformers, drew in his book and occasionally looked out of the window because I told him about something interesting. Well, at least *I* thought it was interesting. Benjamin looked but wasn't at all interested in the lake, the birds or the tall buildings of downtown. He did look a little longer as I pointed out the CN Tower. He remembered it was a cool big building. He'd been up to the top of it the year before when visitors came from England and we did the tour of Toronto. He stared at the tower and sucked in his cheeks, a frown forming across his brow. He was deep in thought.

At Union Station I told him to get his backpack and we headed for the stairs. I wanted to use today to teach Benjamin as much about Toronto as I could but not to make it seem like school work. I had already started home schooling Benjamin so, using the thematic method, I asked him how we could find out where to go next. He pointed to a map on a billboard in the middle of the lobby and we went to check where we needed to go. I told him I had an address so we looked on the map for the street. Once we located the street we looked for the subway line and found the station where we would need to get off. We headed to the subway.

This was the first time Benjamin had been on the subway since he was a baby and safely strapped into a stroller. I wondered how he'd react. If he couldn't handle the travelling, he wouldn't be able to do the work. I prayed every step of the way that day. I really kept God busy! Looking back on it now I realize God was probably smiling the whole time and whispering to my heart.

One day, many years from now, I would finally get it all. Benjamin would be all grown up and it would all have worked out according to God's divine plan. For now, I was just a doubting mother, still at the mercy of people's reactions to my little boy and concerned for his future. I held on tight to his small hand, and knew God was holding mine, and we set off on the next part of the adventure.

After a subway ride and a long walk down the noisy street we arrived at the agency office. Unfortunately, we were a little early. The director, Anne Marie, was sitting at her desk, on the phone. She smiled and beckoned us to have a seat. Oh dear. Benjamin, by now, was getting quite restless. He was fidgeting and making humming sounds, which is what he did when he was getting uncomfortable or anxious. It had already been a long day and stressful for him, and it wasn't even lunch time yet! I told him to get out his note book and draw the subway train. He set to it and I waited as patiently as I could. I was thinking to myself, *"Please let this all be worth it. We still have to travel back home!"*

The director put the phone down and walked over to us. I stood up and shook her hand and I introduced myself. "And you must be Benjamin", she said as she extended her hand. Thank goodness I'd taught Benjamin to shake hands if someone offered their hand to him. He looked at me for approval. Yes, we had talked about bad guys a lot. He wasn't afraid of anyone at this point, but he knew from movies that some people are bad. It was still a concept that troubled him, but thankfully he trusted my judgment. He extended his hand and replied, *"Yes"*, in his robotic monotone, and managed a smile. We were asked to please take a seat at her desk and she started a file for Benjamin.

She asked me a few questions about Benjamin, just general height, weight, age etc. Then she asked Benjamin a couple of questions. His automatic response was to look at me; cheeks sucked in, and hope that I would answer for him. I prompted him a little, but he managed to answer quite well. I was very proud of him. It wasn't very long before he became restless though, and I suspected, quite hungry. I told him to have a seat on the sofa and he could eat his granola bar. I reminded him about the lunch we were going to have at McDonalds in the Eaton Centre and we could go to a giant toy store after too. He sat quietly for several minutes as he chewed and thought about what toy he would buy. They called it bribery back then. I believe the correct term now is 'positive reinforcement'.

The director said we should get some head shots of Benjamin and mail them to her as soon as possible so that Benjamin could start doing auditions for parts, but the snapshots I had taken with me would be fine for background work for now. She said Benjamin was a delightful boy and well-mannered and she was looking forward to working with him. YES! He'd passed the interview and was on his way to being a famous actor!

At this point, Benjamin became restless and couldn't sit still in his seat. He started playing with his *Transformers* on top of the magazines on the table. He was getting louder and the magazines were in jeopardy of being shredded. "Well, I guess the interview's over", Anne Marie said with a big grin. I was so thankful she had a super sense of humour.

Within a few days Benjamin had his first non-speaking role in a movie.

Ok Oscars, here we come!

My endless gratitude to Anne Marie Stewart and *Toronto Casting*, for accepting Benjamin for the unique person he is and for having the foresight to see the possibilities he could bring to the screen even as an autistic eight year old. Thank you for encouraging him every step of the way to 'do that'!

<u>Note:</u> I would encourage every parent, caregiver and teacher, to listen to their autistic child, to any child; not only to their words but also their actions. They're telling us who they are and who they want to become. If you're a praying person, pray that God will guide them to become their authentic self and that you will have the ears and heart to listen. God told Benjamin, not me, who he should be for His glory.

"Even a child is known by his actions, by whether his conduct is pure and right".
Proverbs 20:11

The Big Screen Years

Benjamin's first role in his new acting career was a 'still' role. He played the part of a young boy as photographs on his mother's mantle. It was explained to us as being a retro part. So Benjamin was dressed up in hockey gear with a 50's helmet and 50's skates. It proved quite a challenge as he couldn't skate! Also, the skates were three sizes too big. The assistant director had to carry him onto the ice and try to balance him long enough for the camera crew to take the 'stills'. It took a few attempts but eventually they all managed to take the photos and called it a 'wrap'.

We were both so excited. He got his first paying job as an actor! We celebrated by going to the Eaton Centre to spend his earnings on *'Power Ranger'* toys. At that time, a few hours of work was paid in cash, but more extensive work was paid by cheque or Blue Chips. Most of Benjamin's work proved to be background extra work and covered the GO train and a toy treat on the way home. However, as he got older, he did two projects which proved financially more rewarding.

'The Santa Clause', with Tim Allen, was Benjamin's first lengthy role. He worked over three weeks alongside Mr. Allen and another young actor, David Krumholtz, who later became famous on the hit TV show *'Numbers'*. Benjamin played the part of a painter elf and every day had to go to have his hair and make-up and costume done for his transformation. It was arduous work and I was very proud of his patience. Many days were spent lining up to let assistants paint his face and dress him in colourful costumes that were very hot on sunny August days downtown in an abandoned factory. They pumped air into the building between scenes, but when the cameras were rolling the AC had to be turned off for the sound. The children were all sweaty and tired and red-faced by the end of the day, and 'set moms' were complaining as much as the children. The movie called for a few dozen 'elves' that ranged in age from three years to around fourteen. Benjamin had to wear wool pants, a thick cotton shirt, rubber ears, a felt hat and a long wig. Sweat poured off his face and he became flustered.

One particular scene was troubling for him. He had to polish the sleigh but he didn't do it to the director's liking. Benjamin became very agitated, feeling ashamed and not needed, and walked off the set crying. To my amazement, Tim Allen came over and asked him, "Buddy, what's wrong?" Benjamin told him he was useless at polishing the sleigh. Mr. Allen told him that he too was useless at a lot of things but he kept trying. He asked if Benjamin wanted him to show him how to polish. Benjamin was happy to finally be getting instructions, especially from someone who knew all about TV stuff!

He was particularly fascinated by the mechanics of the 'reindeer'. Some of the crew were excellent with the children and showed them how things worked. Benjamin enjoyed learning about movie-making more than he enjoyed acting, but I was very proud of the way he followed direction and saw things through.

We had a lot of good times on that movie, but a lot of challenges too. Background 'extras' have to put up with a lot, but Benjamin earned enough money to buy his first game and when he was working on set, I became champion parent of the *Game Boy* game, *Tetris*! Benjamin was taught to pay for his expenses out of his earnings. Sometimes there wasn't much left over if he only worked a few hours. We had to take the GO train down to Toronto and quite often a bus or subway train too. After three weeks of filming '*The Santa Clause*', Benjamin bought his Game Boy and a complete set of '*Lion King*' figurines. He was very pleased with himself.

Another movie Benjamin worked on for an extended period of time was '*The Homecoming*', an after-school special with Ann Bancroft. He worked all summer as the stand-in for the lead boy, and bought himself a TV for his room. Part of the money earned, he knew, would be saved for his education. He later used some of that money to publish his first book.

Every opportunity Benjamin had to retreat into his own world, he took. This was his way of calming himself and removing the pressures of being part of a world he didn't feel he belonged to. The pacing came in handy on many occasions where he had to remain quiet but was allowed to walk back and forth. It was also scary when I turned my back and he wandered off. I learned to hold conversations without eye contact, and other mothers would shout, "He's over here!" when we played at the park. Community can be a great support.

A coping strategy that we developed for difficult situations was for Benjamin to walk around an object but not to block people's view or eye contact with someone they were talking to.

On the set of *'The Homecoming'*, Benjamin had to stay where he was told to 'hold'. This was an area designated to the 'extras' and we weren't allowed to wander in case we were called to 'set'. Benjamin needed to pace but the area was too crowded. It was raining and we'd been put in a barn close to the farm house where we were 'shooting'. We were told not to talk or wander off because we could be needed at a moment's notice. There wasn't any space to walk in the barn, so Benjamin, having already learned what to do in these situations placed a bucket the door and began walking in circles around the bucket. It was quite the conversation that night and we had a hard time keeping it down to a whisper. Benjamin wore a path around the bucket and in the morning it looked like aliens had landed in a crop circle!

After *'The Homecoming'* was finished, Ann Bancroft gave the children a large basket of goodies to share. It had candies and small toys in it. Benjamin chose a few candies and – a plastic frog! He still has it to this day.

I was very proud of his perseverance and dedication to his work on the sets. For one movie with Linda Hamilton, he had to get his hair cut very short and shaved at the back, to look like a school boy from the 1940s. He wasn't at all impressed with what they'd done to him, but he was impressed with Linda Hamilton. His only real close-ups during the acting years were for *'FX-The Series'* with Cameron Daddo. He played a delivery boy and got to stand right next to the star with a box of groceries. You can also see him clearly in *'Street Legal: It's a Wise Child'*, and as James Petrie, the young son of a convicted man in *'Scales of Justice'*.

At age fifteen he decided he didn't like to go into Toronto anymore, and so ended his acting career. I was sad in a way. I had enjoyed our times together, travelling on the GO and navigating underground through the shops. But now he was ready to move on to the next 'stage' of his life. He became more independent and finished high school by correspondence at home. His major subject became writing and, through the encouragement of his on-line teachers, he went on to excel at Creative Writing.

The Teen Years

Everybody Line –Up

It's common for children with autism to have a desire (a need?) to line things up. To create unending lines across the living room, kitchen and every available hallway, Benjamin would line up dinosaurs, his chosen fixation during his formative years. They all faced the same direction and were usually specifically grouped, although why they were grouped a certain way changed according to what was on his mind that day. If we were away from home and he was becoming bored, he would line up anything that was handy. This need to constantly occupy his busy mind, far exceeded those early years. Even as a teen, Benjamin would line things up or rearrange them when he became bored.

One day we were in a restaurant and the waitress was taking a particularly long time to come and take our order. Sure enough, Benjamin scouted out the table top and started collecting all the dessert menus, salt and pepper shakers, cutlery etc. His sister owned a bridal shop at the time, so Benjamin began creating a bridal party. There was a salt shaker bride, a peppery groom, a ketchup minister standing behind an upturned sugar bowl podium, and a few seated guests were the sweetener packets. The bride had a deliciously long train made from sugar packets and the menu was the dramatic backdrop for this romantic scene. The entire table was covered by the glorious event taking place until the waitress (obviously a person without any imagination) came and took our orders and left with the backdrop.

This creative scenario drew a few curious looks from those around us and a few smiles and chuckles. Benjamin has always loved that he could make people laugh and, for the most part, he now uses words to convey humour, although I must admit, *Boston Pizza* has had a few strange tables to clear away.

The 'bridal party' took place when Benjamin was around 15 years old. Proof that when we're bored we'll default to what we used to do as a child. Many of us doodle while we're on the phone, some colour in the O's on the programme waiting for the entertainment to start, others will sing to ourselves or conduct an orchestra. You should see Benjamin and me in *Toys R Us*!

<u>Note:</u> So when your child, with or without autism, does something repeatedly, unusual or just plain bizarre, take notice of 'how', 'when', 'where' and 'who' they are expressing in their creativity. It may help you to understand the 'why' someday.

"Before I formed you in the womb I knew you, before you were born I set you apart; ..."
Jeremiah 1:5a

The Rescuer

Although the formative years had been a struggle in themselves for Benjamin, his teen years proved to be a different kind of difficulty altogether. As he watched other boys his age learn to drive and start dating and become independent, Benjamin could only watch and wonder how he could have all these things too; or would he never have them? Most people saw Benjamin as any other teen, not 'different'. He was quiet, withdrawn and mumbled in a monotone voice when he talked, just like a lot of teenage boys. However, unlike most teenagers his age, Benjamin still grabbed hold of my hand tightly when we crossed the street.

Benjamin still had difficulties that became very apparent when he was in public. As I tried to encourage him to be more independent and gain confidence in this world that was still so strange to him, it was increasingly difficult to know when to let go, when to push him a little harder and when to wait. I often had the tendency to try to 'rescue' him from difficult situations.

One incident that was particularly harsh for me was when I asked him to return a movie to the drop-box at the local rental store. I was in another store and could see him from the window. I had parked near the far end of the parking lot and left him with the errand to do alone. I could tell he was nervous but I encouraged him to try and said if he just couldn't do it, he could try again another time. He agreed to try, eager to show he could be 'grown-up'. I watched as he cautiously made his way from our car to the next. He stopped at every car and looked all around. Cars were parked on all sides and some were reversing and others were pulling in to spaces. I knew from his body language that he was getting increasingly upset. I wanting to go out and tell him it was ok, he didn't have to do this. It took all my courage to stand firm and not hold him back from developing his independence.

As I watched him darting through the cars, the woman in front of me turned and said, "He looks suspicious doesn't he? Do you think we should tell the security guard? He may be trying to see if any cars are unlocked". My heart sank. She was right, he looked suspicious; hunched-over, head down, darting from car-to-car with a big frown on his face, but he was trying his hardest to just get through the parking lot and complete the task I'd given him. I didn't want to make the woman feel bad, but I couldn't let her think this about my child, and I wanted people to see that some of us have 'invisible' challenges, whether they are mental, physical, or behavioural.

I told her, *"He's ok. He's my son and he has autism. He's just trying his best to navigate through the cars to get to the movie store. It's his first time trying this. I'm actually very proud of him. He's really not a threat to anyone's car. It wouldn't cross his mind to deliberately do something bad".* Of course she apologized, and I said it was a natural response and I understood. I hope she started thinking about things from a different perspective from then on. I'm sure I would have thought the same as her if I hadn't had a child with autism.

As Benjamin got older he became my 'rescuer' on many occasions. He continues to be my knight and help me in my own battles.

The Young Adult Years

The next few years found us not attending church much. The local churches didn't have youth groups and Benjamin kept pretty much to himself, although he was still working as an extra and found other people who were a little 'different from the norm' on set to talk to.

Eventually, Benjamin became involved in a church youth group in his early teens, and was introduced to girls his age. Everyone in the group was a little awkward as they began the journey of self-discovery and assertiveness. They were finding out who they were and how they fit into the adult world; what they liked and disliked and were making plans for their futures. Benjamin was always delayed socially and more developed intellectually, so he was unsure of the social norms but very aware that he was already mature in his perception of the world. Having a frown on his face constantly because he was concentrating on adapting to the ever-changing dynamics in a social group, and being quiet and reserved as he tried to process it all, he came across as stern and unfriendly. He found it difficult to make friends and even more difficult to talk to girls. They weren't like his sisters and he was simultaneously enchanted by them and unnerved by them.

The youth pastor came alongside Benjamin and they had many long talks about growing up and 'guy stuff'. Stephen (Benjamin's dad), hadn't been able to connect with Benjamin on this level. We learned later that Stephen is probably also on the spectrum, although not as profound as Benjamin. So the neurotypical youth pastor made an impact in Benjamin's life.

The girls in the group tried to include Benjamin in their conversations, as did the boys, once they realized he had social challenges. I was impressed by the care they showed him, but he still felt awkward and unsure with peers. This was something that continued into his early adult years. The youth leader at the church recruited Benjamin's older sister, Anna, to be his assistant, which helped with Benjamin's inclusion into the group. He started going to some of the social events and, although some of them were way out of his comfort zone, he tried his best to participate and the group had patience for him. The youth pastor later became Benjamin's brother-in-law!

After the youth pastor and his bride moved to another town and another church, Benjamin found himself lost again without social interaction. The young people he had come to know were now going off to college and moving away and he was left without friends. Apart from his occasional appearances at his sister's store, Benjamin stayed at home and I became concerned for his social development.

One friend who had stayed in contact with Benjamin proved to be the kind of friend we all dream of having, someone who stays in our life and walks through the mire with us. Shanks is still his best friend today and they've seen each other through some tough times and belly-laughed through numerous TV shows and family gatherings.

God saw our desire to be a part of the fellowship of believers and guided us to a very lively church about a forty-five minute drive from home. We went as guests of Karen's friend. There was a dedication of one of the babies in their family.

What a difference at this church! The people were so friendly and the music was amazing! I recognized the worship leader as the brother of a close friend of mine, so I immediately felt that I had spiritually come 'home'. The pastor was welcoming and funny. I later learned that the church was referred to as a 'seeker-friendly' church. The bulletin said it was "A Safe Place to Find God". I agreed. No pressure to serve the minute they saw us coming; no condemnation, no rules, the pastor even took his jacket off, and in summer the assistant pastor wore shorts! The deciding factor for me was when I read in the bulletin that they had a large youth group. I signed Benjamin up and we met the youth pastor.

He was a young man, not much older than Benjamin who was then 17. He came to Karen's bridal store and met with Benjamin. They went for a walk and talked about 'stuff' and Benjamin came back with a smile. Always a good sign as there were few of them. He was still primarily touting a frown. He said he liked the pastor and so began his adventure with the youth group.

Benjamin was still very quiet and withdrawn but he soon started to attend a Connect Group for male teens. He felt more accepted in this group and made a few friends. The group was led by a married man who had children the same age as the young men, so he was like a father-figure. Benjamin enjoyed talking to him and he even took Benjamin to lunch a couple of times. He knew Benjamin's dad at the time, was quite absent from his life, even though he lived in the same house. The group leader understood this and had a few much-needed, long talks with Benjamin.

As Benjamin outgrew the youth group, and his group leader moved away, he found himself without a Connect Group and unable to make lasting friendships, except for Shanks. So Benjamin and I searched for a ministry to serve in and took a Spiritual Gifts course to see where God had gifted us to serve. We both felt led to the *Alpha* ministry and have since spent several years as part of that amazing group. Watching peoples' lives transformed by faith is a beautiful experience.

At *Alpha*, Benjamin found the acceptance he needed and felt validated as himself, for who he is, not judged for who he isn't. He had support there from the leadership team and prayer partners to share his joys and his struggles. We both felt very blessed.

While we were involved with *Alpha*, we also started a Connect Group at our home. With living so far away from the other participants, Stephen and I hosted the group and served dinner. Benjamin played the video and facilitated the discussion. Although he didn't see himself as being a leader, he led the group through over two years of discipleship. The student had become the teacher. It's now me who goes to Benjamin for scriptural verses and insight into God's character.

It was during the night of *Healing Prayer* at *Alpha*, that Benjamin decided to ask God to bless him as much, or as little as He saw fit, according to His will for his life. Over the next few months, those of us who knew him well saw a gradual change in him. He became more concerned about people's feelings and the ever-present frown was exchanged for smiles. He observed people around him and on TV and started to understand their responses to others. Benjamin became empathic. Over recent years he's been able to help me understand his father better and given opinions on *The Big Bang Theory*. Although he sometimes still struggles with his social interactions at events, his relationships with family and friends have become easier and he's happy to be able to understand people better.

Everyone Has a Purpose

Life Purpose – Mine

We had been learning in church that everyone has a purpose for being here, at this particular moment in history, to further God's Kingdom here on Earth. Through the teachings of the pastors and elders we were encouraged to read Rick Warren's book *'The Purpose Driven Life'*. Benjamin and I also took a course based on Erik Rees' book *'S.H.A.P.E'*, which explains the way God wired us to be the people He created for His purpose. Armed with these two books and a call to action, we decided we would both find out exactly why we were here.

I had recently gone through some changes in my work life and had suffered a deep, long-lasting depression over several personal events which piled up in my life at the same time. I was left without a source of income and very little vision for the future. I was hoping that taking these courses and reading the books would get me back on track and also help Benjamin discover his own purpose.

I must admit, at first I was confused by the whole process and what I discovered didn't seem to make sense as a purpose in my life. At that time I had decided to train as a stager. It was a new-found passion from the TV and I desperately wanted a source of income. My marriage was rocky and I feared it would end in a separation or divorce and I wouldn't have an income to support myself and help Benjamin transition to an independent life. My husband and I eventually rediscovered a friendship in the marriage, so he agreed to pay for my tuition and I started the training.

I thoroughly enjoyed the months of studying and finished my course ahead of time. I had taken the course online because of the distance from the school. However, as I took my final exam, I discovered that the real estate industry had squeezed the staging industry out and had taken over that business, including my school. I was now left with the daunting realization that I would either have to apply for a job as a stager for a real estate firm or start up my own business.

There were a lot of younger, energetic people out there, fresh from school who were pitching for the same jobs. So, I decided to pray about the whole situation and leave it with God. It just seemed like I'd wasted almost half a year and over $1,000 on schooling that promised me work and now was gone. The experience did show me, however, that Stephen was willing to work on our relationship with me. In hind sight, I realize that the training also taught me that I was still able to learn new things but that staging wasn't the career God had in mind for me. Discovering my purpose for Him became the key to my future.

So without a source of income, and Stephen's income at that time just barely meeting all our needs and debt repayments, I went to the Lord again to ask for His will and not mine. Obviously I had been swayed by the TV ads and was not to be trusted with my future! God as always, being a forgiving Father, took me back to the books and His Word and slowly opened my eyes to the person He had created in me. He took me back to the things I had loved as a child and the heart I had as a child. Slowly, I began to realize who Lynne was.

Among other things, as a child I had loved to garden with my great-uncle, Tom. He used to take me to a small community plot where he would teach me how to grow vegetables. Also, I had been excited to visit the tiny yard of my great-aunt, Pat, and she would show me her pet turtle that lived in a clay pot turned on its side, next to a bucket of water dug into the ground which served as his pond.

I remembered the words of my dear grandparents too, that I was such a kind and giving child, I would give my last sweetie away. This is the Lynne that God created before life happened and got me off track. I didn't feel like that person anymore, but God is merciful and has all the time in the world to take us back to the beginning and start over from there. So, I gave my future to Him and asked Him to lead me on.

The result was a gardening business which took a few beatings due to a knee injury. I gave up after a year, thinking I couldn't do it anymore and I must have heard God wrong - again! I had enjoyed my gardening business immensely and was terribly upset at letting it go. Moreover, it had provided a small amount of income for my daughter too and I was hoping we could work together, along with Benjamin. I had hoped it would become a retirement income for me and Stephen too. We would still have a mortgage at retirement. So, as I got depressed again and felt like a complete failure, (the enemy knows too well, our weaknesses), I asked God again what on earth was happening in my life.

He took me back to a realization I'd had in my teens. As a person who wanted to help others, I had started nursing school but been forced to leave when my parents moved, (long story. Maybe this is the idea for another book?).

During my nurse's training, however, I discovered I was drawn to psychiatric care. I had left nursing behind because of moving and traumatic changes in my life, but God reminded me that life had put that desire aside, not Him. So I asked Him what He wanted me to do with that now. He reminded me of a course I had taken as a Christian counsellor but had put on hold to home school. Well, they tied in, so I pursued that thought and decided to go back and brush-up on my training.

After extensive searching online I realized the course I had taken years before was only for an assistant and not a full counselling course. Apparently, I would have to be male and an ordained minister to complete their course! So I searched for a school where I could train online and finish my diploma and set up office, without a sex change. Dismayed, I ended up looking for an alternative to the $7000 the schools were asking for classes, plus the need to leave home for 3 years. The courses were not a good fit, either. I wasn't sure why, just sure that these were not for me.

I finally found a course online that sounded perfect and would allow my earlier training to count towards a new career in Life Coaching. This was a great fit for me. I wouldn't have to leave home, it didn't cost a lot and I would be taking people from where they are now in their lives to move forward with positive goals in mind. No sex change required.

As part of my training, I needed at least six volunteers to be my first clients, and a practising Life Coach to be my mentor. As it so happens, (as God so happens), I had gone to a Life

Care Centre to seek assistance with these new changes in my life so that I wouldn't lapse into another depression. I was determined to stay on track with God. We'd come this far, I needed to see it through and actually 'get it'. The person I had been recommended to was herself a Life Coach and was happy to be my mentor. At the time of this writing, she is still my mentor and now good friend.

So I enlisted my first few volunteer clients and had amazing success with helping them find their Life Purpose. By this time, Benjamin had already discovered what God was calling him to do with his life, so I asked him if he would try life coaching with me to see if it lined up with what he already knew to be his calling. It did! I was overjoyed. Benjamin was a little more subdued but elated that I had finally found *my* calling.

Note:

When we pray and get a "No' from God, it may be because the prayer is:

"...either not good in itself, not good for us or for others, directly or indirectly, immediately or ultimately". (5)
- John Stott

This is a poem that I read often and memorized as a young child, while rocking in my Great-Aunty Pat's kitchen:

"I shall pass through this life but once.
If, therefore, there be any kindness I can show,
Or any good thing I can do,
Let me do it now;
Let me not defer or neglect it,
For I shall not pass this way again."
-Stephen Grellet

Benjamin explains in his book, *'My Life A.S. Is: An Inside Look at Autism and Asperger's Syndrome'*, how he came to discover God's plan for him, so I won't rewrite it here.

However, I will tell my side of his story about his first publication, 'The Kingdom', in my next chapter.

Life Purpose – Benjamin's

Benjamin had written his first book for publication. He had written a rough draft of another book but had decided to wait to publish that. He had started attending the annual writers' conference organized by *The Word Guild,* which presents the opportunity to read new work in a group of other aspiring writers and published authors. They liked his work and encouraged him to have it published.

Having a limited income at the time, he decided to enter his manuscript in a writing contest, hoping his work would be accepted well enough to win a mention and subsequent discount on having his book published. To our delight, *'The Kingdom'* was well-received and placed him on the honour role. He had earned a discount to publish his book and the book would be on the Great Canadian Authors list!

After many months of emails and late nights and nervousness, Benjamin's first book was published. We celebrated with family and friends at our local *Boston Pizza*, which has become our restaurant of choice for all our celebrations since the 'Salt and Pepper Wedding Party'. Benjamin read from his book and even had his picture taken for the local newspaper.

I watched my son, now a grown man; being accepted by his peers in the life God had called him to live, being embraced by family, friends and strangers as he realized his dream. The struggles and heartaches had finally brought the person Benjamin is to the fulfilment of his Life Purpose as a Great Canadian author.

Benjamin went on to write his autobiography, *'My Life A.S. Is – An Inside Look at Autism and Asperger's Syndrome'* about growing up on the autism spectrum, and is currently working on other books. I hope he will publish many more books and keep encouraging parents and inspiring other young adults on the spectrum to reach for their dreams. I am so very proud of him.

When people meet him for the first time now, they still say he's quiet, introverted and polite. When they get to know him, they say he's hilariously funny and quirky. If they give him a title, it's usually Artistically Eccentric. Not bad for an autistic kid.

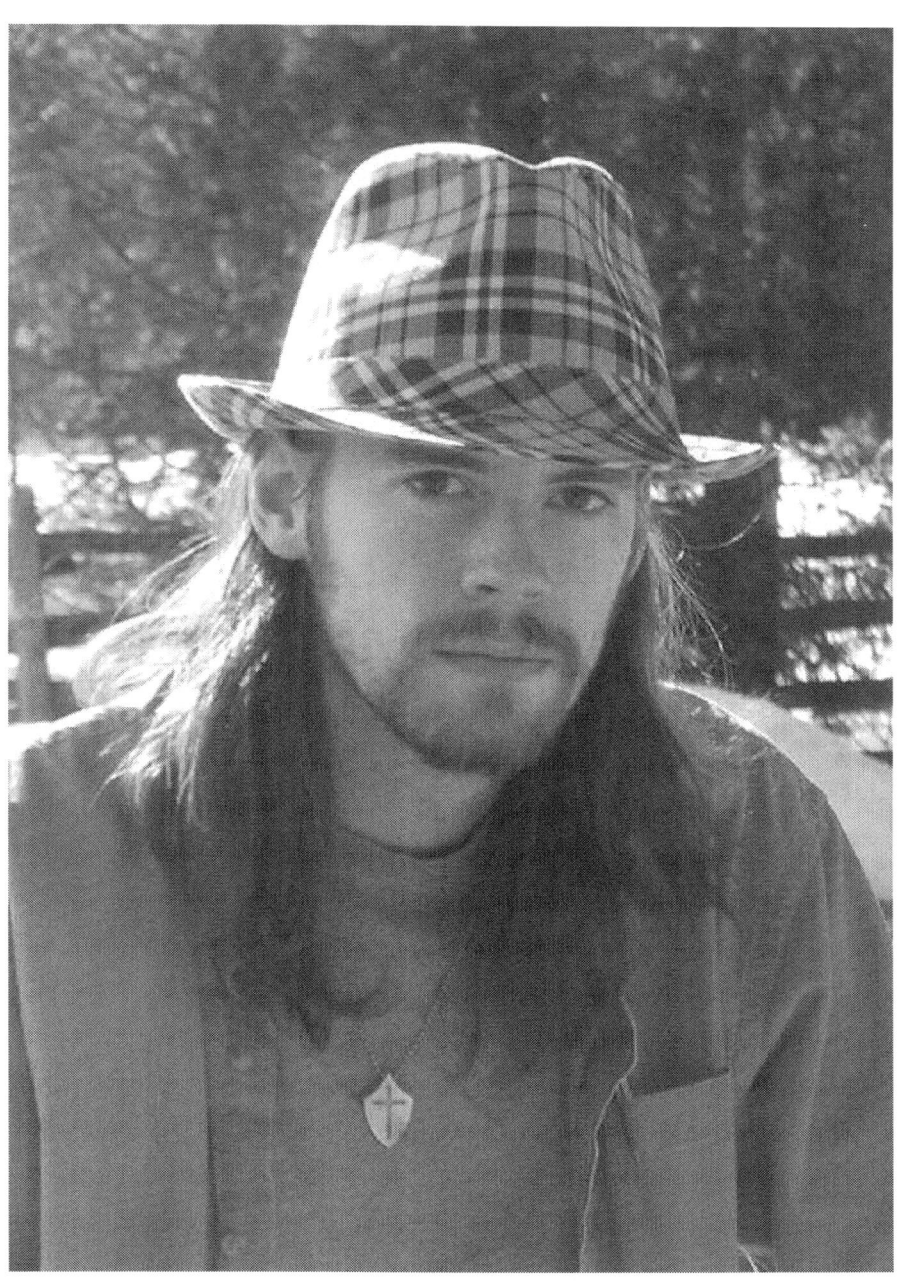
Benjamin at 27. Published Author.

The Journey

People say, "It must have been difficult, raising an autistic child". I tell them,

"*No, it wasn't difficult. Other people made it difficult sometimes; but for me, it's always been an amazing journey*".

Look,
Look into my eyes my little child.
There,
There you are.
This is where you go to, my Sunshine;
Into a world you created with God,
To find the man you'd become;
To tell your own story.

I used to sing this song to Benjamin when he was small and it's still *his* song:

"*...Be courageous and be brave, and in my heart you'll always stay forever young...*"

'Forever Young' by Rod Stewart

About the Author

Lynne grew up in the small town of Keighley in England. She still loves anything Victorian, mushy peas and fish & chips, and teaching her grandchildren "true English". In her teen years she immigrated to Canada, and married Stephen at the young age of 19.

She became a mommy at just 20 years old, and spent most of her youth chasing after her three children – Anna, Karen and Benjamin.

Now a grandmother to four boys (Josiah, Elijah and Nate here earth and Caleb in heaven) and one girl (Kara Lynne), Lynne still loves to spend time with the children in her life.

Lynne has a knack for making people feel special – be it a birthday celebration, a home decor makeover, brewing someone a cup of tea, or taking time to sit and chat – you are always better off for having known her.

Gardening is a new love of Lynne's, as well as writing and self-publishing. As she gets older, she is discovering more of who she is than ever before.

Mum - it is glorious to watch you bloom. You are still teaching us kids how to live life to the fullest

-Written by Lynne's oldest daughter, Anna

Footnotes

1 Benjamin T. Collier. *My Life A.S. Is: An Inside Look into Autism and Asperger's Syndrome* (Winnipeg, Manitoba: Word Alive Press, 2013) p91

2 Benjamin T. Collier. *My Life A.S. Is: An Inside Look at Autism and Asperger's Syndrome* (Winnipeg, Manitoba: Word Alive Press, 2013) p76

3 Benjamin T. Collier. *My Life A.S. Is: An Inside Look at Autism and Asperger's Syndrome* (Winnipeg, Manitoba: Word Alive Press, 2013) p75

4 Benjamin T. Collier. *My Life A.S. Is: An Inside Look at Autism and Asperger's Syndrome* (Winnipeg, Manitoba: Word Alive Press, 2013) p82

5 Nicky Gumble. *The Alpha Course Manual: An Opportunity to Explore the Meaning of Life; quoting John Stott* (Deerfield, IL: Alpha North America,1993) p19

6 Continental Hair
Benjamin grew his hair long because he wanted to help others but didn't have a lot of money. He chose to do what he could that didn't have a monetary cost – grow hair and donate it to an organization that makes wigs for children who have lost their hair through cancer treatment.

continentalhair.com

Recommended Reading & Other Material

The Holy Bible – God's Word

'My Life A.S. Is: An Inside Look at Autism and Asperger's Syndrome'
by Benjamin T. Collier
published by Word Alive Press; Winnipeg, Manitoba

'The Kingdom'
by Benjamin T. Collier
published by Word Alive Press; Winnipeg, Manitoba

'The Purpose Driven Life'
by Rick Warren
published by Zondervan; Grand Rapids, Michigan

'S.H.A.P.E'
by Erik Rees
published by Zondervan; Grand Rapids, Michigan

'Wild at Heart'
by John Eldredge

published by Thomas Nelson Inc; Nashville, TN

'Captivating'

by John and Stasi Eldredge

published by Thomas Nelson Inc; Nashville, TN

Alpha.org

'The Alpha Course – An Opportunity to Explore the Meaning of Life'

by Nicky Gumbel

published by Alpha North America

'Star Trek: The Next Generation' (TV Series)

Darmok and Jalad at Tanagra: Episode 2; Season 5

Some Mothers Do 'Ave 'Em (BBC Series, on YouTube)

Starring Michael Crawford and Michelle Dotrice

Have a Break, Take a Husband. March 8, 1973

Books by Benjamin T. Collier

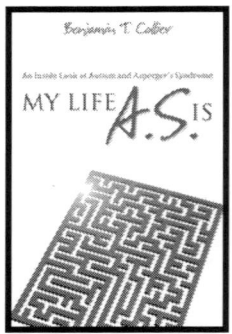

'My Life A.S. Is: An Inside Look at Autism and Asperger's Syndrome'

Benjamin T. Collier

'Autism and Asperger's Syndrome continue to affect an increasing number of children and adults around the world. They are puzzling conditions that create a barrier of communication between the child and anyone who wishes to know what the child is experiencing.

After twenty-plus years of living on the Autism Spectrum, Benjamin T. Collier has written this book to help families understand a part of what their autistic loved ones may be going through'.

"Benjamin gives his readers a unique glimpse into the world of Autism from the viewpoint of one who's lived there. He writes honestly about his experience growing up on the Autism Spectrum *while engaging the reader with his distinctive sense of humour. With a non-neurotypical mind, Benjamin challenges his audience to view the world from a different perspective..."*

Merry C. Lin

PhD, CPsych. Clinical Director, LifeCare Centres

Available from: WordAlive Press and Amazon

ISBN: 978-1-77069-778-2

Or for an autographed copy, email Benjamin:

benjamintcollier@thewhiterosewriters.com

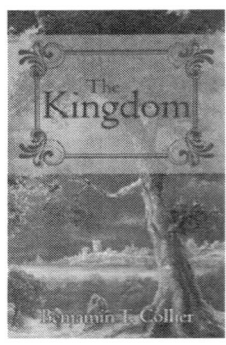

'The Kingdom'

Benjamin T. Collier

'The Kingdom of Allandor, once ruled by a noble king who vanished years ago, now lies in the hands of a corrupt steward. In her chambers, Princess Nevaeh, daughter of the king and heir to the throne, waits endlessly for a man whose heart is noble enough to take back the kingdom with her, but no such man can be found. In the dead of night, an unlikely invader into the kingdom sets events in motion which could alter the fate of the kingdom forever'.

"Benjamin Collier... (is) a special person, a gifted writer with an explosive imagination... His inspired words carried me into worlds and adventures far beyond my experience. When you open the cover of 'The Kingdom', hold tight to your chair but release your imagination as Benjamin transports you on flights of fancy".

Ray Wiseman

Author, columnist and recipient of The 2009 Leslie K. Tarr Award.

Available from: WorldAlive Press and Amazon

ISBN: 978-1-77069-219-0

Or for an autographed copy, email Benjamin:
benjamintcollier@thewhiterosewriters.com

NOTES

Made in the USA
Charleston, SC
19 March 2014